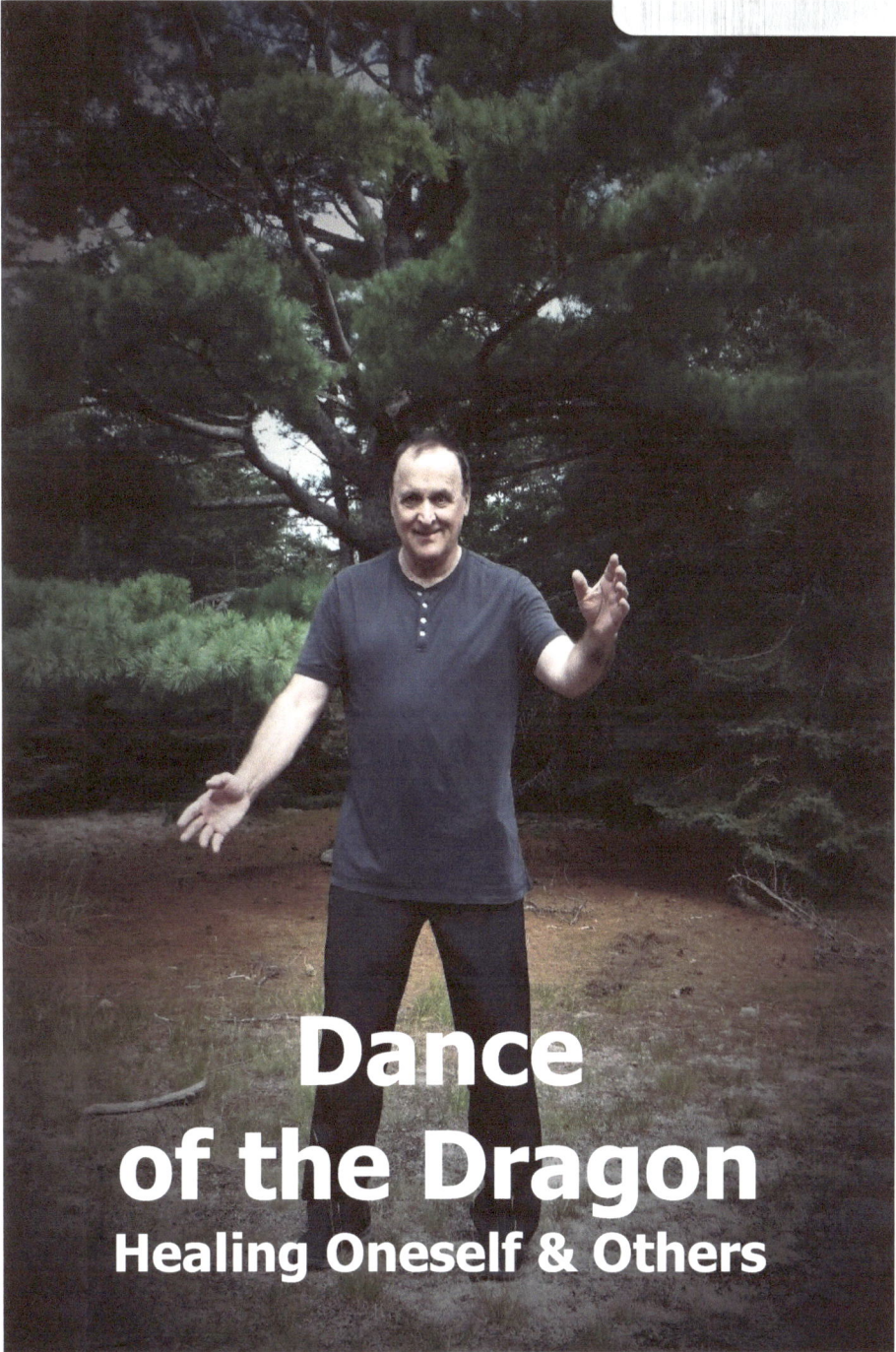

Dance
of the Dragon
Healing Oneself & Others

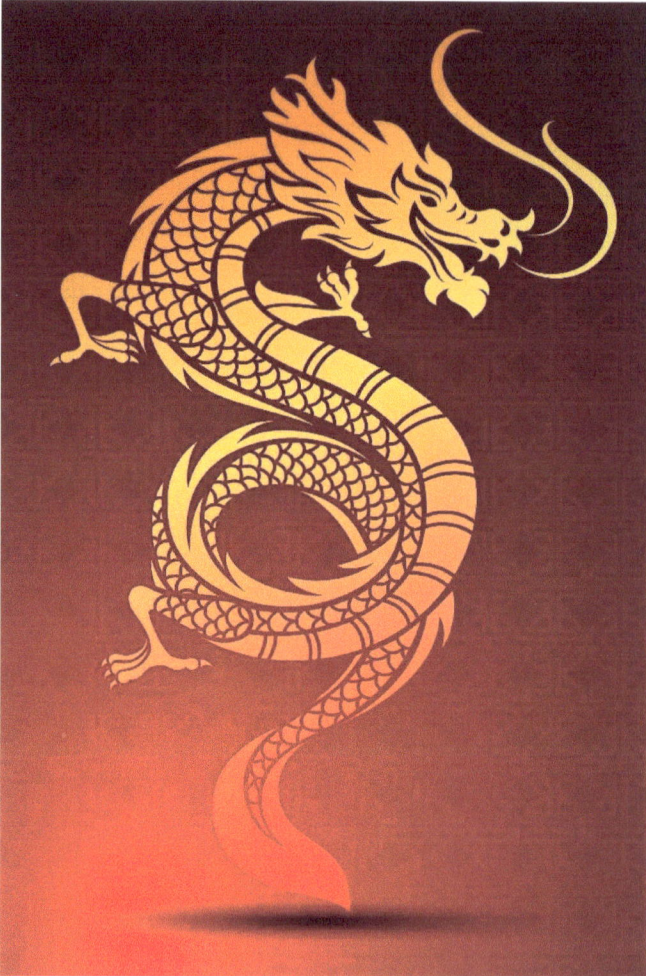

In Chinese philosophy, the Qi that moves between the physical and spiritual realms is often referred to as the Dragon. Chinese dragons are gentle, friendly and wise. They embody strength, wisdom, and luck. They have domain over both fire and water.

Dragons are also a symbol of healing. In Chinese medicine, practitioners may work with the internal and external Dragons when there is a disconnect between body, Mind and Spirit. In the context of this publication, the dragon symbolizes the ability of the healer to dance or move freely with the chaotic nature of the Universe to rebalance the Qi of the patient.

Table of Contents

Qi Gong for Self-Healing

Qi Gong for Healing Others

Preface

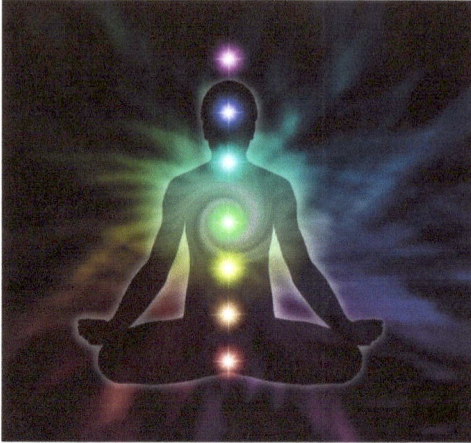

Qi Healing is one of the most powerful treatment modalities available to humankind. Some people are born with a natural ability to heal others with Qi or Universal energy. With the proper training, most of us have the potential to provide effective Qi Healing treatments by developing the special functions inherited at birth such as knowing the future or the past, seeing auras, seeing energy along the body's meridians or energy pathways, and seeing inside the body.

In China Qi Healers work in hospitals alongside traditional medical doctors. In some hospitals in North America nurses offer Healing Touch with the approval of the patient's doctor. Reiki, a Japanese form of Qi Healing, has become very popular in many North American communities.

Independently of the style of Qi Healing, there are common principles that govern its expression as an art and a science. Qi Gong Masters stress the importance of self-healing. To heal others, one must embark on a personal healing journey and learn to let go of emotional and energetic blockages that impede the abundant flow of Qi.

The main ingredient of Qi Healing is strong and vibrant Qi. Having a kind and compassionate Heart is central to developing strong Qi. Disciplined practice of exercises to clear, build and balance Qi is a basic requirement of being an effective Qi Healer.

A Qi Healer's energy needs to be strong to overcome pathogenic Qi. Otherwise, toxic Qi may infiltrate the healers body only to manifest itself over the years physically and spiritually as disorder and disease.

Energy is information. Students of Qi Gong learn not only by the spoken word but also by a transfer of energy-information from the instructor to the student. The palms are the antennas that capture the energy-information transmitted by the instructor.

Qi Healers can feel, see, or sense the energy of another person thus initiating a transfer of information. As palms scan a body, they can feel the other person's energy directly. Some Qi Healers can see another person's energy emanating from the chakras, acupoints, meridians or aura. Energy-information can also be transferred instantaneously from one person to another as energy spheres intertwine.

Conditions must be right for the transfer to occur. Listen to your body to become aware of the energy transfer. The body is relaxed and rooted, the Mind is clear, and the Heart open.

The Qi Healers main diagnostic tool is to listen from the Heart, open and receptive, without judgement. To access these special functions Qi Healers must first listen to their own bodies and embark on their personal healing journey to balance and refresh their own Qi.

Understanding the concepts of Qi is only the beginning. Only through regular practice of Qi Gong, mindful movement, breath and meditation will true knowledge emerge of the Power of Qi.

This publication provides a theory of natural healing. It contains information gathered from many teachers, notably Qi Gong Masters Weizhao Wu and Tsu Kuo Shih. It is beneficial to receive training from an experienced Qi Healer to receive the direct transmission of information from teacher to student via the informational source that represents Qi.

This book details Qi Gong exercises for self-development. It also provides exercises to learn how to see, feel and move Qi. Several basic diagnostic techniques are explained in addition to some powerful Qi Healing methods. Finally, a section on how to deal with toxic Qi provides some insight on how to stay healthy while helping others rid themselves of pathogenic Qi.

But more importantly it offers two major Qi Gong forms to explore and integrate universal Qi. One style develops the ability to feel and build strong Qi in the palms. It also trains the Mind to move the Qi. The second style trains the practitioner to move Qi in the major acupoints, the Micro and Macro Cosmic Orbits, in the Shu and Mu Points, and in the 12 Regular Meridians.

Both forms develop strong Qi in the Lower Dantian.

Finally, a road map is provided to help Qi Healers treat others in a safe and compassionate environment. The Universe thrives on chaos. To be an effective Qi healer, learn to Dance with the Dragon and move with the ever-changing energy landscape that presents itself to us every day of our lives.

About the Author

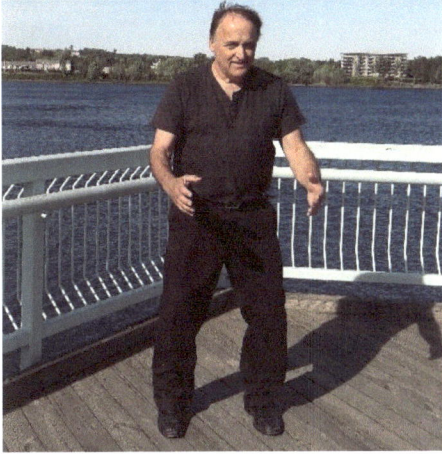

Maurice Lavigne has been studying various aspects of universal energy via the martial and healing arts since 1971. He first heard about Qi in the early 70s from a martial arts teacher who published weekly commentaries on Qi in a local community newspaper in his home town of Bathurst, New Brunswick, Canada.

He studied the martial arts of Jui Jitsu and Shotokan Karate for a total of six years before enrolling as a student of Aikido, a Japanese art of self-defence. In 2013, Maurice was promoted to the rank of 4th Dan by Osawa Hayato Shihan of Japan, Technical Director of the Canadian Aikido Federation.

"Aikido's approach to self-defence is unique in the martial arts," Maurice said. "Its powerful techniques are based on the ability to relax, center and blend with aggressive behavior. A positive attitude and sense of compassion favors the unification of one's Qi with the Qi of the Universe. This self-defence art is challenging to master, as it requires an open Heart and the letting go of our innate desire to control the outcome of events."

Maurice was first introduced to Qi Gong in 1987. Since then he has been fortunate to study with two accomplished masters of the art: Master Weizhao Wu of Wu's Qi Gong and Tai Chi Fitness Center in Toronto, Ontario, and Grand Master and Doctor of Chinese Medicine, Tsu Kuo Shih, of the Chinese Healing Arts Center in Danbury, Connecticut, USA.

Since becoming a student of Qi Gong Maurice has received Certification in many styles of Qi Gong and Tai Chi from Master Weizhao Wu of Toronto as well as Certification as a Qi Healer from Grandmaster Tsu Kuo Shih of the Danbury, Connecticut.

During his years of training in Qi Gong, Maurice became a Registered Massage Therapist. He pursued his interest in Energy Healing and Acupressure Massage by studying various energy healing modalities such as Cranial Sacral Therapy, Reiki, Healing Touch, and Oriental Pressure Point Therapy.

Maurice has also received certification as a Yoga Instructor from Fitness New Brunswick and has developed a unique style of Yoga called Restorative Qi Yoga featured in his second book on Qi Gong called Qi Gong's Five Golden Keys.

In 2009, he was awarded a Diploma in Advanced Acupuncture from the College of Acupuncture and Therapeutics of Kitchener, Ontario, and in 2013 Certification as a Chinese Herbalist from the Institute of Chinese Herbology of Concord, California.

Maurice practices Acupuncture, Massage Therapy, Herbology, and Qi Healing at the Fredericton Wellness Clinic Inc in Fredericton, New Brunswick, Canada, where he also teaches Qi Gong classes and workshops.

He is the author of five books: The Power of Qi for Health and Longevity, Qi Gong's Five Golden Keys, Dance of the Dragon - Healing Oneself and Others, Acupuncture Diagnostic Methods and Point Selection, and the Acupuncture Fertility Handbook.

The Importance of Virtue

Like many things in life, true understanding of Qi comes with experience. Learning Qi Gong exercises allows us to travel where others have travelled before and to experience what they experienced. It provides a foundation for developing strong Qi and enables us with proven Qi healing methods.

Some Qi Gong healers live longer lives than others. Several factors determine the longevity of a Qi Healer. Hereditary factors play an important role. We are all born with a potential that can be developed to a degree. Exposure to environmental toxins, unhealthy diet, and injuries can limit our potential. Emotional factors play an important role.

What are the secrets of longevity? According to my former teacher, Grand Master Tsu Kuo Shih of Connecticut, USA, to achieve longevity one must:
- Calm the Mind with no thoughts. Drop down to Center
- Cultivate life energy or Qi
- Live a life of Virtue: Love, compassion and respect

Energy comes from food and air, and before that, from the Universe. Everything is Universal Energy. We are too. You can gather and store what you need by the practice of Qi Gong.
All energy has a Yin/Yang component which must be balanced for the body to be healthy. If the Qi flows freely you enjoy good health and wellness. If Qi is blocked and the body is not balanced for an extended period, you may get sick.

Although many different situations can break the Qi such as negative thoughts, environmental factors, and an unhealthy diet, emotions play a key factor. By cultivating a calm Mind and a compassionate Heart, by helping others, you will be happy all your life.

According to Grand Master Shih, in order to acquire Qi, one must be kind and give from the Heart. Jealousy takes energy. It is very bad for you. Powerful energy comes from doing good. Do good for others. Live according to the laws. Be happy and peaceful. Great virtue is easy. Believe and it will be so!

Types of Qi

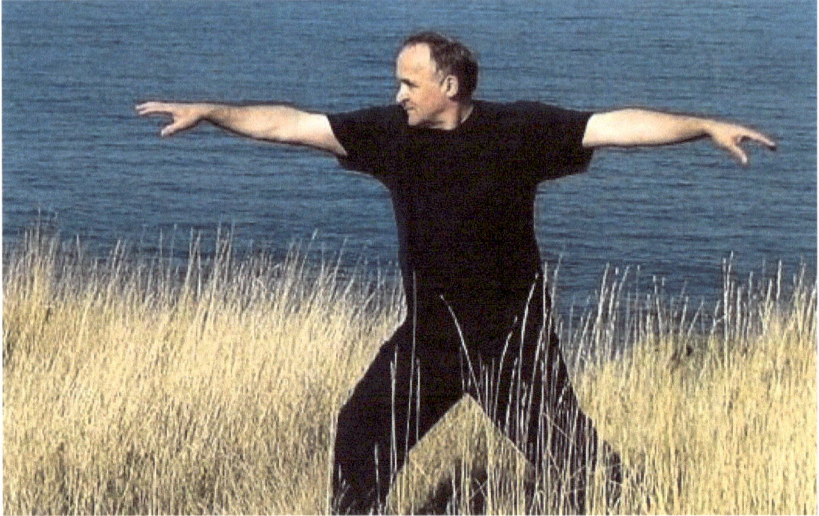

Qi can be described according to the function it fulfills in the body. The following are a few types of Qi, the understanding of which may be useful in the practice of Qi Gong.

- **Jing or Essence** is derived from one's parents and is supplemented by acquired Qi. It is responsible for growth, reproduction and development, is stored mainly in the Kidneys, and circulates all over the body, especially in the Eight Extraordinary Meridians.

Kidney Jing produces Marrow. The Brain in TCM is called the "Sea of Marrow". Therefore, if Kidney Jing is weak, the brain may be undernourished, leading to such symptoms as poor memory or concentration, an "empty" feeling in the head and dizziness. Weak Jing in children may lead to poor bone development, slow learning and poor concentration. Weak Jing in the elderly may lead to deafness, osteoporosis and unclear thinking.

- **Yuan Qi or Original Qi** is derived from Jing. It can be viewed as "Jing in motion". It promotes and stimulates functional activities of the organs and provides the foundation or catalyst to produce Zhen or True Qi. It originates in the Ming Men or Gate of

Fire, circulates via the Three Dantians, and pools in the meridians at the Yuan Source points.

- Kong Qi or Air Qi originates from the air received by the Lungs.

- Gu Qi or Essence of Food and Grain Qi originates from the transformation of food by the Spleen in the Stomach. The Gu Qi rises to the chest where it combines with Kong Qi (Air Qi), floats down like mist from the Lungs onto the other organs below and passes to the Heart where it is transformed into Blood.

- Ying Qi or Nutritive Qi nourishes the organs and helps to produce Blood. It circulates in the main meridians in a 24-hour cycle and flows with the Blood in the main meridians and within the Blood vessels. This aspect of Qi is needled with acupuncture.

- Wei Qi or Defensive Qi helps to protect the body, warms the surface of the body and regulates body temperature by opening and closing the pores. It is found on the surface of the body and within the muscles and skin, but not within the meridians. Its circulation is dependent on the Lungs.

Qi Functions and Disharmonies

Qi supports vital functions within the body. When a disorder arises, it is a disruption in the function of Qi. A prolapsed organ, for example, is a disruption in the ability of Qi to provide the raising and stabilizing function on an organ. A frontal headache with emotional instability may point to stagnant Liver Qi. Bilateral lower back pain could be the result of weak Kidney Qi. The main functions of Qi within the body are:

- **Transformation:** Qi assists in the formation and transformation of fundamental substances within the body into vital energy, for example the transformation of food into Qi and Blood.

- **Transportation**: Qi is the foundation of all movement and growth in the body.

- **Protection:** Qi defends the body from external pathogens.

- **Raising and Stability:** Qi holds the organs in place, keeps Blood in the vessels, and governs the removal of fluids.

- **Warming:** Yang Qi of the Kidneys and Spleen warms the body.

Whenever the movement of energy is blocked, disorders in Qi function occur. Qi has **four main states of imbalance**. These imbalances may affect many parts of the body at once such as a meridian or an organ system.

- **Qi Deficiency:** May affect the Lungs with symptoms of shortness of breath, or the Stomach and Spleen with poor appetite, fatigue and weakness. The primary treatment needed to rectify a Qi Deficiency condition is to tonify the Qi.

- **Qi Stagnation:** May affect the Liver and lead to chest or hypochondriac pain that is not fixed in location. The primary treatment needed to rectify Qi Stagnation is to move or regulate the Qi.

- Sinking Qi: Sinking Qi may affect the Spleen and lead to digestive issues and prolapsed organs. The primary treatment needed to rectify Sinking Qi is to raise and supplement the Qi.

- Rebellious Qi: May affect the Lungs or Stomach and lead to coughing, belching, vomiting, hiccups or dizziness. The primary treatment needed to rectify Rebellious Qi is to calm and subdue the Qi.

Jing, Qi, Shen

Jing, Qi, Shen form the essential trinity of our physical manifestation. They continually interact mutually supporting each other.

Jing Qi is determined at birth by our genetic makeup. It is the underlying physical essence, a mixture of constitutional or genetic force that is associated with the sexual function and vitality of a person but without the clearly obvious active energetic presence of Qi. It is often associated with the perception of depth or a quality of endurance of a person. Jing creates form.

Qi is the vital active force that animates the physical body and its vital functions. It is a person's vitality that causes others to describe them as energetic and alive. A person may have a strong Shen or mind, but their body may not be very vital or alive. When the body has Qi, the person is obviously energetic. Excessive sex, worry, negative emotions, stress, over work and thinking deplete Qi.

The combination of Jing and Qi nourish the Shen which is generally translated as the Spirit-Mind that forms the active force for maintaining form and providing consciousness. When it is disordered, the form of a person changes and consciousness becomes disturbed.

Using Qi Gong, we can build the Dantian energy, situated in the lower abdominal area, producing more Jing Qi Shen. By putting the Mind in the Lower Dantian, with a relaxed body and tranquil Mind, without desires and thoughts, energy will come.

Just place the Mind there naturally until it feels warm or full. Resting the Mind in the Lower Dantian waters the seeds of Qi creating the potential for development and growth.

Three Dantians

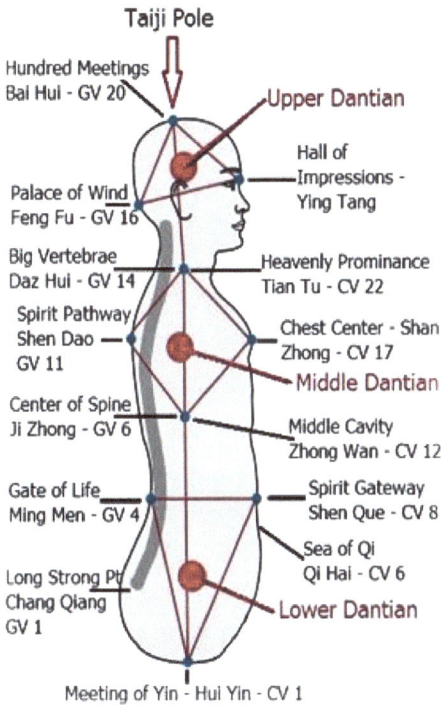

Taiji Pole

Hundred Meetings
Bai Hui - GV 20

Upper Dantian

Hall of
Impressions -
Ying Tang

Palace of Wind
Feng Fu - GV 16

Big Vertebrae
Daz Hui - GV 14

Heavenly Prominance
Tian Tu - CV 22

Spirit Pathway
Shen Dao -
GV 11

Chest Center - Shan
Zhong - CV 17

Middle Dantian

Center of Spine
Ji Zhong - GV 6

Middle Cavity
Zhong Wan - CV 12

Gate of Life
Ming Men - GV 4

Spirit Gateway
Shen Que - CV 8

Sea of Qi
Qi Hai - CV 6

Long Strong Pt
Chang Qiang
GV 1

Lower Dantian

Meeting of Yin - Hui Yin - CV 1

According to Medical Qi Gong, humans have three important energy centers called the Upper, Middle and Lower Dantians. A Dantian or Elixir Field is where Qi is gathered, stored and transformed.

The Three Dantians communicate with each other via the Taiji Pole. This energetic channel flows from the Bai Hui point on the crown of the head, through the center core of the body, to the center of the perineum at the Hui Yin.

The Three Dantians connect smaller energy gates called Chakras, or spiraling wheels of energy, that originate from the Taiji Pole and spiral outwards into the body's energy field.

The Lower Dantian or House of the Earthly Realm is the center of physical strength and stamina. It is here that Yuan Qi originates and resides. This Dantian is in the lower abdomen in the center of the triangle formed by joining the point located at the navel called Shen Que or Spirit Gateway, the point on the lower back called Mingmen or Gate of Fire, and the center of the perineum called Hui Yin or Meeting of Yin.

The triangle faces downward allowing the Lower Dantian to gather denser Yin energy from the Earth. Earth energy is required to help ground the Qi Gong practitioner, balancing the active Yang energy gathered during the practice of Qi Gong. Collecting energy in the Lower Dantian increases awareness and intuitive perception leading to naturally occurring body movements.

This zone is primarily responsible for physical strength, sexual vitality and overall health. Qi Gong practice encourages returning to the source or Lower Dantian to help strengthen the root of the body's energy.

The Middle Dantian or House of the Human Realm gathers lighter less substantial Yin and Yang energy from Heaven and Earth, creating a distinct kind of emotional energy normally associated with human beings. This reservoir for mental and emotional energy reflects the Heart's energetic capacity to express feelings and show compassion. It is associated with storing Shen or Spirit, with respiration, and with the health of the internal organs, in particular the thymus gland. Its energy is more akin to vibration.

The Middle Dantian's field of energy naturally extends into both palms. It is the main region responsible for the refinement of vitality or Qi into Spirit. It is located at the level of the Heart in the mid chest area. It forms a square with its four extremities defined by six acupuncture points.

Its lower front point is located on the abdomen half way between the navel and sternocostal angle called the Zhong Wan or Middle Cavity. The front center point of the Middle Dantian is located at the center of the chest, on the midline of the sternum called the Shan Zhong or Chest Center. The upper front point of the Middle Dantian is located at the suprasternal notch called the Tian Tu or Heavenly Prominence.

The upper back point is located above the 1st thoracic vertebrae called the Daz Hui or Big Vertebrae. The mid back point is located above the 6th thoracic vertebrae between the scapula called Shen Dao or Spirit Pathway. The lower point is located above the 12th thoracic vertebrae called Ji Zhong or Center of Spine.

The Upper Dantian or House of the Spirit Realm collects energy from the Universe - Sun, Moon, Planets and Stars, and represents your spiritual aspect. This energy is more akin to vapor. It is associated with light and is Yang in nature. It is the least substantial of all three energies. This is where the wisdom Mind perceives subtler vibrations and frequencies emitted by the earth, planets and stars. Psychic perceptions and intuitive knowing that transcend time and space emanate from this region.

The center of the Upper Dantian is in the pineal gland, a small endocrine gland, located near the center of the brain between the two hemispheres. The pineal gland produces melatonin, a hormone that affects the modulation of wake/sleep patterns and photoperiodic (seasonal) functions. Mystical traditions and esoteric schools have long known this area in the middle of the brain to be the connecting link between the physical and spiritual worlds.

The Upper Dantian is shaped like a pyramid facing upward. This allows it to gather energy from the Stars. It transforms Shen into Wuji or the openness of infinite space.

The front gate of the Upper Dantian is located at the center of the eyebrows called the Yin Tang or Hall of Impressions, the back gate in a depression immediately below the external occipital protuberance called the Feng Fu or Palace of Wind, and the highest gate is located at the top or crown of the head called the Bai Hui or Hundred Meetings.

The combined energetic qualities of all three Dantians form the foundation for all psychic perceptions. Pure intent and a quiet Mind are required to favor accurate psychic perceptions and true communication with the higher self.

Each Dantian collects energy from the Universe and redistributes it to all the internal organs. In turn, this energy is projected into the body's Wei Qi field. **Wei Qi** *(pronounced "whey chee")* translates as **"protective energy."**

In Traditional Chinese Medicine, the Wei Qi field is limited to the surface of the body, circulating between the skin and the muscles. In Medical Qi Gong, the Wei Qi field includes the three external layers of the body's subtle energy fields sometimes referred to as the body's Bio-Energy Field or Aura.

The Wei Qi field surrounds, flows through, and extends from the human body. The energy from the Lower Dantian projects about an inch away from the body into the physical field, the Middle Dantian projects to about a foot and a half away from the body in the emotional field, and the Upper Dantian projects several feet away from the body in the intuitive or spiritual field.

Foundations of Qi Gong Energy Healing

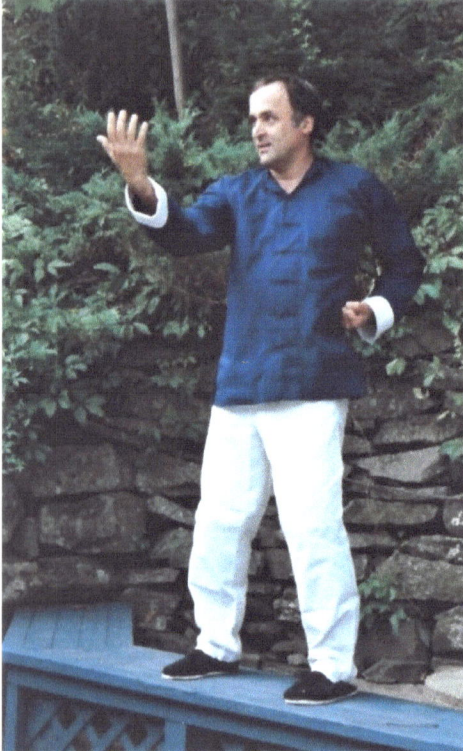

Qi Gong (chee-GONG) is the current name for what was formerly known as Taoist breathing exercises that date back nearly 5,000 years.

Qi means energy, the energy of the Universe. Gong means to gather with skill. Therefore, Qi Gong can be defined as a disciplined practice to gather energy from the Universe with practiced skill.

There are over 3,000 forms of Qi Gong. The three major schools are medical, martial and spiritual. Qi Gong uses posture, gentle, slow, rhythmic movement, breath, mental imagery and mindfulness to clear out stagnant Qi and gather universal Qi into the body. The results calm the Mind, energize the body and help to create a sense of balance, both mental and physical.

Qi can represent space, air, breath, or the vital life force – it depends upon the context with which it is used in a sentence. Qi Gong is a method to attract, gather, store, balance, cleanse, and guide Qi for various purposes.

In doing so Qi Gong develops balance, both physical and energetic. It fosters health and well-being for yourself and others, as well as longevity, strength and agility, intelligence or wisdom, and spirituality.

Foundation Elements

- **Body Posture**
- **Body Movement**
- **Breath**
- **Mind Moving Qi**
- **Mindfulness**

Body Posture

All Qi Gong work begins with good posture. When the body is properly aligned energy flows more abundantly. The objective of good posture is to allow the bones of the skeleton to stack up one upon the other in perfect balance thus allowing the body to stay upright with little or no effort. The energy thus liberated can be used to strengthen the flow of Qi and to promote good health.

The following guidelines may help you gain the sense of good posture in your own body. Remember these are only guidelines. Good posture starts at the feet, the body's foundation.

Relax, letting the weight of the body flow downwards towards the center of the earth, while maintaining extension upwards through the Crown Point on the top of the head. Develop deep roots. Relax and keep your Spirit up. Stillness increases Yin energy.

Qi Gong can be practiced standing, sitting and lying down. It can also be practiced walking or running. Regular practice strengthens the Qi Healers energy allowing the practitioner to provide a more effective and safe treatment.

Standing

- Stand in an upright position, feet shoulder width apart, weight 70% on the heels to develop Yin energy or 70% on balls of feet to develop Yang energy
- The Bai Hui or Crown Point is aligned with the Hui Yin located in the center of the perineum which is aligned with the line joining the heels or the balls of the feet
- The Crown Point touches the sky

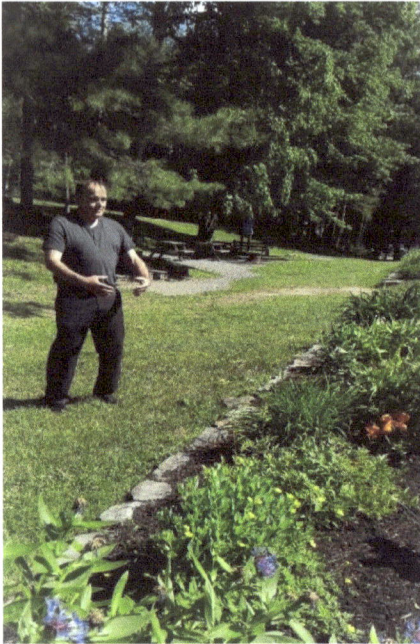

- Look far to the horizon. Keep the eyes soft and open, or half closed
- Gently let the chin move inwards and up towards the Adams apple
- Place the tip of the tongue on the palate behind the front teeth
- Gently close the anal sphincter
- Let the arms hang down and slightly away from the sides of the body
- Gently press the abdomen to the inside of the lower back. This will tilt the hips forward, straightening the lower back
- Keep the knees straight but soft. Never lock the knees
- Keep the feet rooted deep into the earth
- Rest the Mind in the center of the abdomen

An erect spine and stable lower body structure help the body resist the constant pull of gravity. This benefits the overall energy of the body by reducing the activity level of the muscles involved in maintaining upright posture. It reduces resistance to the flow of Qi, improving overall health and wellbeing.

Standing meditation is more beneficial after 40 years old. Sitting too long can lead to High Blood Pressure, lower back and hip pain, and circulatory problems in the lower body. Standing meditation helps grow more energy more quickly in the Lower Dantian than sitting.

Sitting

When sitting on a chair, always sit on the edge of the chair to help open the Hui Yin located on the pelvic floor between the reproductive organs and the anus. This ensures that the chair does not restrict the reproductive organs.

Follow the general indications for standing. In addition, the lower legs are perpendicular to the floor, palms facing up resting on the mid thighs on the distal head of the ulna bone. Keep the arms rounded and maintain a space the width of your fist at the armpits. If you suffer from back pain it is advisable to rest the upper body on the inside back of the chair.

Remember that palms facing upward raise blood pressure, and palms facing downward lower blood pressure. Palms facing up allow you to receive energy from the teacher and the Universe. Palms facing down encourage a deeper sense of relaxation.

Sitting in Hero Pose or in a Lotus or Half Lotus posture helps build Dantian energy and facilitates the movement of energy in the Micro-Cosmic Orbit.

Lying-Down Method

Practice the Lying-Down Method before and after sleep, after walking, or at the end of a Yoga or Qi Gong class. Do Whole Body Breathing or Relaxed Belly Breathing explained later in this publication. These exercises relax the body and build energy.

On the Back: The head rests on a 4" pillow or yoga block to open the back of the neck. The hands rest on the sides of the body, palms facing the body. Keep the Bai Hui or Crown Point open.

On the Side: Lay on the right side (left side could be harmful to the Spleen, Stomach, and Heart). The right arm is bent, with the thumb near the right eyebrow. The left hand rests on the side of the body below the hips. The right leg is straight. The left leg is bent to help with balance. The Ming Men or Gate of Fire is open and the belly is relaxed. This is like a drawn-bow posture. Practice Relaxed Belly Breathing.

Advantages of Good Posture
- Less pain
- Muscles are relaxed
- Body is open
- Qi flows
- Opens energy doors at joints
- Favors circulation of Blood and Qi

- Helps to relax the body and move the Qi
- Develops positive emotions
- Helps to focus the Mind
- Helps to connect with the earth
- Develops balance
- Three-point alignment with the Tai Chi pole allows for standing with less effort as the bones are stacked one upon the other with little muscular effort
- Facilitates body movement

Body Movement

Together with posture, repetitive movement activates the circulation of Qi and Blood by mechanically squeezing stagnant Qi and Blood from blocked areas. Qi tends to stagnate at areas of the body that contain muscular tension. Repetitive movement facilitates a systemic rebalancing of the Qi by relaxing muscle tension and facilitating the flow of Qi through the channels.

Body movement also harmonizes the body's nervous system and increases the flow of lymph and intracellular fluids. The lymphatic system is very low-pressure system. It relies upon muscular contraction to move the lymphatic fluid. It is therefore important you move unless you have physical limitations at which time the extent of movement may be determined by your physical capabilities.

Elements of Good Movement
- Unbroken
- Soft
- Flowing
- Supple
- Good rhythm
- Shifting weight
- Inward and Outward
- Opening and Closing

Advantages of Good Movement

- Improves the flow of energy
- Moves interstitial fluids
- Increases the pumping action of Blood and the lymphatic system
- Opens meridians favoring the flow of Qi
- Increases Yang energy
- Harmonizes the nervous system
- Focuses the Mind
- Develops coordination and balance

Breath

Breathing is the first thing we do when we leave the security of our mother's womb and the last thing we do before we die. Breath allows for an exchange of Qi with the Universe. On exhalation, toxic energy leaves the body and moves into the Universe. On inhalation, new fresh energy comes to the body.

Proper breathing increases the intake of oxygen, massages internal organs, cleanses the body, calms and centers the Mind, unifies Body and Spirit, supports the gathering, moving and release of Qi, and leads to a deep state of relaxation.

Breathing brings oxygen into the cells of the body and helps cleanse the body of toxins. It massages the internal organs making them healthier and encourages proper posture. The organ's functions become stronger.

Observing breath calms the Mind, harmonizes the body, and encourages the flow of energy or Qi. Still the Mind and relax the body. There should be no thinking, or the body will be tight.

Breath and energy are one. In Traditional Chinese Medicine (TCM), the Lungs govern the Qi and respiration. They disperse or move the Qi through the entire body via the energy channels and their collaterals. The Lungs cause the Qi to descend to the lower part of the body, activating and fueling the vital physiological functions associated with digestion and the formation of Blood.

The Lungs also rule the surface of the body and the Wei Qi, or protective Qi that, according to TCM, moves just below the surface of the skin, and according to Qi Gong theory expands a few feet outward from the body. The Wei Qi forms a protective barrier to the invasion of the body by external pathogenic factors such as Heat and Cold.

Breathing Methods

There are various breathing methods practiced in Qi Gong depending on the desired results.
- Natural Belly Breathing for relaxation
- Reverse Belly Breathing to strengthen Qi
- Varying Length Breathing (Longer inhale to build Qi - Longer exhale to encourage relaxation)
- Pulsating Breath (To harmonize the Heart beat with the breathing rhythm)
- Double Exhalation or Double Inhalation (Accentuates the effects of inhalation or exhalation)
- Pausing the breath on inhalation (Builds more Qi) or on exhalation (Deepens the relaxation response)

Elements of Good Breath

- Breath from the abdomen
- Breathe in and out through the nose for relaxation
- Relation breathing is silent, soft, deep, continuous, slow but comfortable
- For increased relaxation, listen to the tranquil space at the end of exhalation letting the inbreath rise on its own
- With physical exertion breathe in through the nose and out through the mouth, or in and out through the mouth

Mind Moving Qi with Direction and Intent

Everything is composed of the same energetic substance called Qi. Although energy may appear to take on different forms, energetically everything is interconnected as one body. This subtle energy or Qi manifests itself as the visually obvious physical body.

The Mind leads and controls the Qi and the Qi directs the essence or Jing. The Mind directs Qi or vital energy which draws the Jing with it. In practical terms, the Qi follows whatever the Mind focuses on. The Mind leads the Qi to a certain place.

When the Qi is focused there and gathers the essence, substance will be formed. Physical change will occur. Using the Mind to move and rebalance the Qi is the most powerful form of Qi Healing.

In the beginning students of Qi Gong use visualization to help move the Qi. With practice they begin to feel the Qi between the palms, in the meridians, and lower Dantian. Over time the practice of visualization leads to consciousness awareness of the flow of Qi in oneself and others.

The following are two methods that help understand the concept of Mind leading the Qi.

1. Finger Lengthening and Shortening Method

This method helps train the Mind to move the Qi. It helps you to learn to use the Mind to affect physical change. From a sitting position, measure the length of the fingers by placing the palms together using the crease at the wrist to properly align the hands.

Place the palms facing up on the thighs. Relax and imagine for a few minutes that the center finger of one hand is getting longer. Feel that hand getting full while the opposite hand feels open. Then measure the length of the middle finger again using the same wrist crease as a base to see if you were able to lengthen the targeted finger.

2. Meditating on a Problem Area

In the presence of an ailment such as an ache or pain that has a specific and definite location meditate on that area to facilitate healing. This encourages the Qi of the body to move to the affected area to rebalance the flow of energy and reduce pain.

First look within the affected area. Inhale with awareness. Exhale and relax the area. As you exhale allow any uncomfortable sensations to disappear.

Then using the Mind, bring Qi to the area. If there is too much Heat, imagine a cooling or reducing effect. If there is a too much Cold, imagine warmth moving to the area. If there is an imbalance, imagine a rebalancing or normalizing of the Qi.

Mindfulness

Mindfulness has been defined as a mental state achieved by focusing one's awareness on the present moment, while calmly acknowledging and accepting one's feelings, thoughts, and bodily sensations. Mindfulness has become a household word in some North American communities. It is a very positive remake of meditative practices that have been around for thousands of years.

Qi Gong focuses on mastering form and movement. Combining breath with movement unifies the body and the Mind further intensifying practice. Add visualization techniques to allow the Mind to move Qi in the meridians and energy centers and Mindfulness becomes a launching pad to mastering the movement of Qi.

As in any discipline, a student of Qi Gong first learns basic techniques to be able to eventually move to a higher level of understanding of Qi. With sustained practice students begin to feel the presence and movement of Qi in their bodies and in those of others. Once they have reached this level, they can use the Mind to unblock stagnant Qi, build strong Qi and rebalance the body's energy.

Some people have a natural ability to feel the Qi. Women feel Qi more readily than men. A small percentage of people will never feel the Qi.

Most develop a conscious awareness of the presence of Qi as a natural progression of sustained practice. Mindfulness helps students of Qi Gong become consciously aware of the Qi in oneself and others raising the efficiency of practice and creating more powerful Qi for Healing.

Six Keys to Qi Healing

According to one of my beloved teachers, Grand Master T.K. Shih, to be a good Qi Healer it is important to understand the Six Keys to Qi Healing.

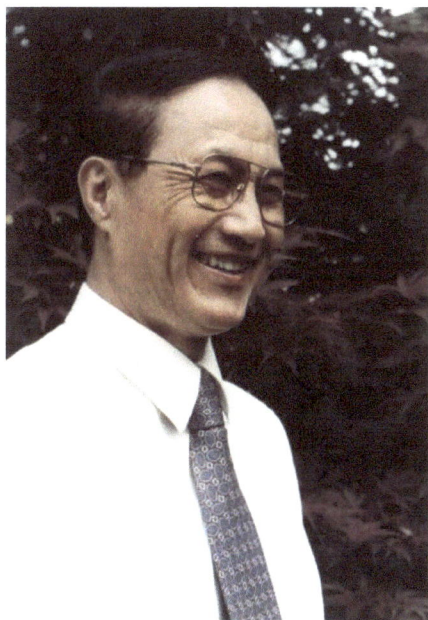

1) Mind Has Power

Understand that Mind has power. Intention directs Qi. If there is pain in part of the body, put the Mind there and energy will follow. Use the Mind to re-establish energetic balance and to create and affect reality. Even at a distance energy can function because the Mind has power.

Qi has many qualities. It is instantaneous. Distance is of no importance. It can go through metal. Qi is not bounded by time or space.

This Key is the most important as it makes the difference for a Qi Healer between success and failure. Understanding this guarantees you will be a good Qi Healer.

2) Body is a Precision Biological Instrument

The body is a precision biological instrument which can be open to receive, send, maintain or expand energy. You can turn the energy on or off at will switching it on for Qi Healing and respect of others. The instrument becomes more powerful with disciplined training and by being harmonious and polite.

3) Different People, Different Special Functions

We all have different roots. Different people, different bodies function differently. People can have different special functions. Each person has something special that they can do that not everyone else can do. You need to be open to look for you special function and find it. Once you become aware of your special function or functions, with practice you will develop them further.

Special functions are often repressed by society. They get lost in our perception of how life should be lived. Special functions are different from person to person as the roots of wisdom differ. Training with a Qi Gong Master and meditation can open special functions.

Examples of special functions are long distance healing; precognition; knowing the future or the past; seeing auras; seeing the energy in the meridians; seeing inside the body; smelling distant fragrances and hearing distant sounds.

4) Different people, Different Sensitivity to Qi

Everyone has a different sensitivity to energy. Some feel energy immediately, some feel energy only after lengthy practice, and 5% never feel energy. Some may feel Qi in some training methods and not in others. They can still be a good Qi Gong practitioner, but teachers and healers must feel the Qi.

If a person does not feel the Qi, he/she should continue to practice as over time most people will feel the Qi. More practice brings more healing, more energy and more sensitivity to Qi in oneself and others.

5) Different People, Different Temperaments

Different people have different temperaments. Some control others and are leaders. Some are controlled and are followers. Some people, however (one in a hundred) can't do either. They don't control their own bodies and should not practice with energy.

Others need scientific proof before they believe. To understand the nature of Qi these individuals should keep an open Mind to facilitate learning.

It is important for a Qi Healer to know their patients. Different patients have different personalities: Some are natural adapters. They learn quickly and are flexible. Others are technology minded. They need to know the details of how everything works.

Some have a scattered Mind. They need help to relax and focus. And others have a controlling Mind which breaks the Qi.

We are all individuals and it is fine to be different. Ultimately each person is responsible for their own healing. A healer needs to master different methods to be able to heal different disorders and to satisfy different temperaments.

It is important to gain the trust of patients by being good to them. In return patients must respect the healer. If the patient is not comfortable with the healer, he or she should be referred to another practitioner.

6) Qi is Inside the Words

Words are like seeds. When planted, they will grow. Words can heal.

Learn to listen not only with the ears. Keep the hands open and receptive to the words of the patient. Be positive, frank, honest and open. When showing respect your body will be open to receive the patients words and energy-information. Only then will you know what to do to help the person. Always speak from the Heart as words can heal.

Written words also have energy that can be sensed. You can sense words on paper with the hands.

Points to Remember when Practicing Qi Gong

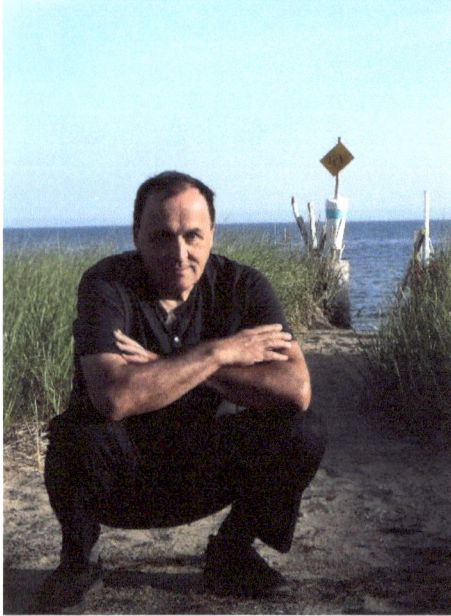

Find a good place to practice with lots of fresh air. Where you practice and the people who are in that place affect the quality of the practice. You need a space that is quiet with good energy. Find where you belong, which trees you feel better with. It is good to always practice in the same location as it builds energy in that space.

Important points to remember:
- The quality of the environment affects the quality of practice
- Practice in a quiet and peaceful place, with lots of fresh air
- Oxygen is essential for the body to survive
- Energy will build in this place
- Body will feel very good

Avoid rain and wind because when the pores of the body relax they open making it easier to get a cold. The back and spine have a lot of acupoints that are connected directly to the organs. The feet are doors to the earth, so it is easy to catch cold from the feet. There should be no wind from the back or the feet.

Wind from the front is fine as it is not easy to catch cold. Wind to the head is fine as it moves from the head down the outside of the arms and massages the body. Do not practice Qi Gong in thunder and lightning as the overcharged atmosphere may disrupt the flow of Qi in the body.

Five Point Evaluation Method

There are many Qi Gong schools – Medical, Buddhist, Confucius, Taoist, Martial Arts... To be effective, the method must be right for you or it will not work. If it does not work for you, it is not your method. You may not be able to practice a lot of methods.

To be a Qi Gong Healer, you must be able to choose the appropriate method and respect the following five points for effective practice:

- Proper Body
- Proper Breath
- Proper Mind
- Proper Direction of Qi
- Proper Intention of Qi
(Dredge/Reduce, Smooth/Regulate, Gather/Augment)

Good Person/Good Heart

Mental attitude is extremely important. Develop a good Heart. Do good for others. Play a positive role in society. Respect others. Do not lie or be angry. Bad deeds accumulate negative Qi in this life and possibly in the next.

Be kind. You must want to help people and do good in the world. Make things right with your family and friends. Change your thinking about people who you can't help. Correct yourself every day. Even the highest person must cultivate a good Heart.

- You must truly want to help others
- Never say another person is bad
- Be selfless
- Speak from the Heart
- Being happy helping others opens the door to good energy
- Respect friends, parents, family, and teachers

Roots of Wisdom

Before learning Qi Gong, the door to your special functions may be closed. Qi Gong opens the door, revealing special abilities that were there from birth. Keep your Mind open. Trust the wisdom of Qi Gong and the special functions will open.

Your roots come from your biological conditioning through your genes, essentially from your parents. The roots provide the special functions such as knowing distant events and seeing energy. You cannot choose your roots, but you can make good roots for the next life.

Get to know yourself and your special talents. Be smart about your special talents. Special functions require special roots which you will become aware of in the future with disciplined practice of Qi Gong.

Profound Understanding

Allow yourself to understand at a profound level. If you understand at this level, the knowledge is yours. Be calm, peaceful and relaxed. Keep the Mind open. Use the Mind to develop:

- Sudden Understanding
- Knowing from the Heart

Anywhere, Anytime

Practice in any order, anytime, anywhere, but follow the basic principles. Practice with consistency and perseverance.

- The more you practice the more energy you have
- Qi Gong becomes part of everyday life
- Be happy with everyone
- Mind quiet and peaceful
- Correct body and breath
- Speak good about others. Make them look good. Help make people healthy and lucky

This publication introduces a very high-level Qi Gong. There are enough methods to practice 24 hours a day. As it is impractical to practice 24 hours a day, follow the principles of Qi Gong while you are doing other things.

Try to practice three times a day. From 3 to 5 a.m. is a powerful time to practice. Also, before lunch, then at night before bed. The Stars and the Moon are present two of the three times. During the early morning and at night more of the Universe is visible since our atmosphere is not radiant with the Sun.

The direction you face, the time you practice, the place where you practice can make a difference but are not crucial. Just remember to practice!

Qi Healers 15-Style Form

This form helps Qi healers feel and build strong Qi in the palms. It also strengthens the ability to use the Mind to move Qi. Many of these exercises can be used on others in a Qi healing session.

1. Open with Universe Meditation

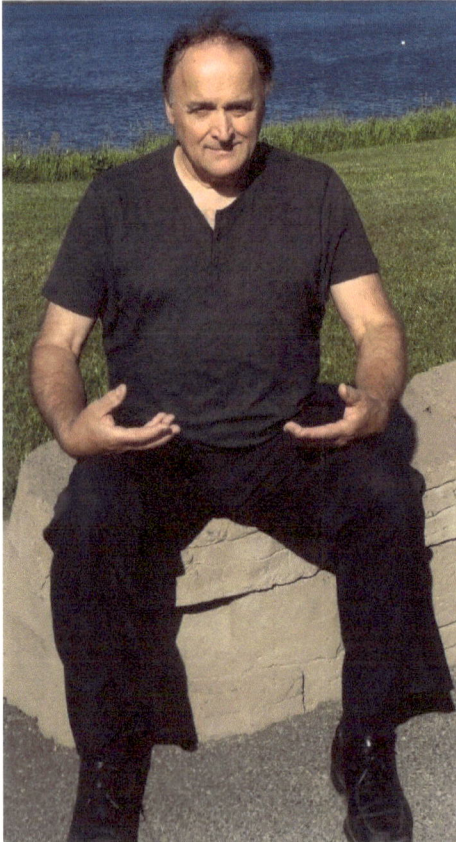

Open with the Universe Meditation is often done at the beginning of practice to relax the body and focus the Mind. When in a class setting, the teacher will often send out Qi to the group and energetically tune the students.

The first six exercises in this form can be done sitting or standing. When sitting place the back of the wrists on the thighs, feet shoulder width apart, and lower legs perpendicular to the ground. Sit on the edge of the chair or bench to allow the free flow of energy in the Micro Cosmic Orbit. Gently close the anus and place the tip of the tongue lightly on the palate behind the upper teeth.

Relax the body side, front and back, head to toes, one section at a time: Line 1 = Side of body from Yin Tang to Middle Fingers; Line 2 = Front of Body from the face to the big toes; Line 3 = Back of the body from the back of the head to soles of the feet.

Line 1: Mid Eyebrow Point; Sides of Head; Shoulders; Elbows; Wrists; Fingers; Middle Finger

Line 2: Face; Throat; Chest; Abdomen; Reproductive Organs; Pelvic Floor; Hip Joints; Knees; Ankles; Toes; Big Toes

Line 3: Back of Head; Upper Back; Mid Back; Lower Back; Tail Bone; Back of Knees; Heels; Soles of Feet (Yong Chuan - Gushing Spring)

For a deeper relaxation, spend more time at the Mid Eyebrow Point or Yin Tang - Hall of Impressions.

On inhalation expand the part of the body you are focusing on outward as big as the Universe. On exhalation relax and let go. Be open with the Universe. Smile from the Heart. Universal energy will come to you.

After doing the three lines one to three times, on inhalation, expand the whole body outward as big as the Universe. Imagine the Universe is within you. Expand every cell out to the Universe, then every molecule, photon and particle. Every cell is filled with Universal Energy. Relax on exhalation. Repeat each level 3 to 6 times.

The body grows bigger, as big as the Universe. It's a big Universe. Be open with the Universe and its planets, moons, stars, galaxies, and endless open space. Be happy and relaxed with the Universe. The Universe is you! Smile from the Heart. Smile to every cell. Smile to the Universe. Open the Heart. Universal energy will come to you. Toxic energy get out! Shoot out! Good energy, universal Energy come in! Smile to the energy!

Meditation is important as it opens your natural healing abilities. This builds Jing-Qi-Shen. To help your patients you need strong Jing-Qi-Shen.

To finish place the palms over the Lower Dantian, bringing Qi to the abdomen, men left hand first, women right hand first. Relax the Lower Dantian. Put your Mind in the center of the abdomen. The Mind is in the Dantian, but not in the Dantian. Cultivate no thoughts! Be peaceful. Energy will grow. Keep your energy, Universal energy, and the master's energy in the Lower Dantian.

2. Eight Diaphragm Abdominal Breathing

Four major diaphragms, located in the center core of the body, work together in unison to contribute to the respiratory rhythm which is fundamentally important for the proper functioning of the central nervous system, circulatory system, and critical metabolic / systemic functions.

The palms of the hands and arches of the feet may also be considered as diaphragms. Although they may not be directly involved in breathing, they are important in receiving and extending energy or Qi, the breath of life.

- Pelvic Diaphragm

The pelvic diaphragm is located at the pelvic floor and is important in the elimination of solid and liquid waste (the downward and outward movement of Qi from the body).

- Respiratory Diaphragm

The respiratory diaphragm, the most common and well-known diaphragm, separates the thoracic cage from the abdomen. It is located at the base of the Lungs, massages the internal organs and aids in breathing.

- Thoracic Outlet Diaphragm

The Thoracic Outlet is comprised of the first thoracic vertebrae T1 called the Big Vertebrae, the first ribs and manubrium, the upper part of the sternum which attaches to the clavicles, and the cartilages of the first pair of ribs. The Thoracic Outlet diaphragm is composed of the tongue, the muscles of the hyoid bone, and scalene muscles. It helps control breathing and speaking.

- Cranial Diaphragm

It is well documented in Osteopathic studies that the Central Nervous System (CNS) has a certain "rhythmical motion" to it called a Cranial Sacral Rhythm. In other words, it has life and pulsates to mobilize Cerebral Spinal Fluid (CSF).

This rhythmical movement is said to be intimately linked to the cardiac rhythm and is profoundly affected by breathing patterns.

The cranial diaphragm is composed of differentiated connective tissue in the skull called the Tentorium Cerebelli. The tentorium separates the cerebellum from the inferior portion of the occipital lobes.

The diaphragms are related to each other anatomically and therefore, functionally. Their function must be maintained to prevent symptoms of pain, congestion of fluid, dyspnea or shortness of breath, and other disorders.

When you consider Breath and Qi as synonymous, the palms of the hands, soles of the feet and front thoracic and abdominal region of the body may also be considered as diaphragms involved in the exchange of energy with the Universe. At a deeper level each cell may be considered a diaphragm as their movement facilitates the exchange of fluids and energy with the immediate environment.

The Eight-Diaphragm Breathing exercise combines Relaxed Belly Breathing with visualization to move the eight diaphragms. This breathing method helps release tension in all three Dantians or energy centres and harmonizes the Triple Warmer or San Jiao which is composed of three parts, the Upper Warmer which controls intake, the Middle Warmer which controls transformation, and the Lower Warmer which controls elimination.

Some medical researchers believe that the Triple Warmer is associated with the hypothalamus, the part of the brain which regulates appetite, digestion, fluid balance, body temperature, heartbeat, blood pressure, and other basic autonomous functions. The Eight-Diaphragm Breathing also trains the practitioner in the pushing and pulling of Qi from the palms and soles of the feet.

This technique can be practiced sitting or standing. When in a standing posture, move 70% of body weight back to the heels. Then raise the hands to the height of the Middle Dantian and hold with relaxed belly breathing.

Belly Breathing is practiced throughout most Qi Gong forms, except when an alternate form of breathing is required, as it helps relax both the Mind and the body making the practice more effective.

Inhale through the nose, to the count of seven, expanding the lower part of the body, front, side and back. Exhale through the nose to the count of ten letting the chest drop down. Repeat 10 to 30 times. The breath is gentle, silent, slow, deep and unbroken. Let the inhalation rise on its own from the space between exhalation and inhalation. Thirty breaths equal about five minutes.

Now add the dropping the four diaphragms on inhalation combined with relaxed breathing. As you inhale visualise the pelvic floor, respiratory diaphragm, thoracic outlet diaphragm and tentorium drop. On exhalation the four diaphragms naturally return to their relaxed position.

Once you feel comfortable with moving the four diaphragms add the diaphragms in the palms and soles of the feet to your practice for a total of eight diaphragms.

3. Stretching the Qi

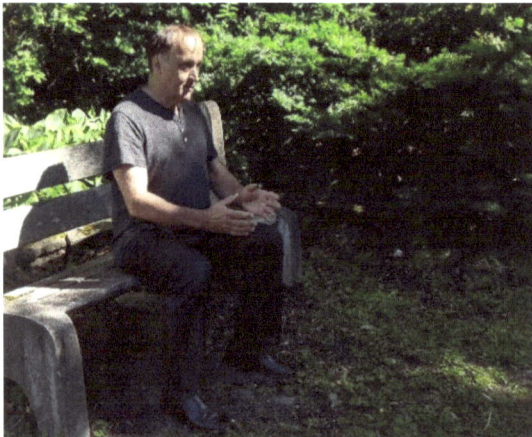

The following exercise helps develop greater sensitivity to Qi. The center of the palms are aligned. The palms face each other about two fists widths away from the lower abdomen. To start, palms are nose width apart. Look far into the distance. Focus the attention on the center of the palms which can be seen in the peripheral vision.

Inhale with Belly Breathing expanding the palms to head width. Exhale returning to the nose-width position. Repeat 6 to 9 times.

Inhale expanding the hands outward from head width to the width of the shoulders. Exhale and return to the head-width position. Repeat 6 to 9 times.

Repeat the previous exercise but once you reach shoulder width, vibrate the palms back and forth three times before exhaling.

Exhale and return to the head-width position. At the end of the exhalation vibrate the palms three times. Repeat 6 to 9 times.

4. Grinding the Qi

After stretching the Qi horizontally, hold an energy ball in front of the navel palms facing each other, head width apart. Grind the Qi by rotating the hands much like the pedals of a bicycle being aware of the Qi sensation between the center of the palms. Spin the Qi starting slowly, increasing speed as you progress. The hips may vibrate naturally from side to side releasing tension in the lower back.

Focus the mind on the center of the palms. Move as fast as you can comfortably. Rotate 300 times then place palms on the lower Dantian for a few minutes to consolidate the Qi.

5. Turning the Qi Stick

This exercise gathers Qi from the Universe. It is as though an energy or Qi stick extends from the Lao Gong or Palm Center into the center of the Lower Dantian. As you turn the stick around, you are turning energy around which will flow centrifugally into the Lower Dantian like water in a drain that has been spun, building Dantian energy.

The left hand is resting along the side of the body if you are standing or on the left thigh if sitting. Place the right hand about a fist width away from the lower abdomen. Palm is facing the abdomen. When you feel an energy connection and warmth, make circles or spirals in a clockwise direction for men and a counterclockwise direction for women.

Gradually increase the speed and the diameter of the circles expanding outward for 300 turns. Then reduce the spirals for 300 turns. The movement must be circular to develop a lot of Qi. Don't go into boney structures, such as the rib cage, xyphoid process or pubic bone. Feel the energy spiraling around the whole body while only circling the hand around the Lower Dantian. End with a decrease of speed and diameter of circles.

Slow down to a stop. Place the hands on the Lower Dantian, men left hand under right, women right hand under left. Hold the Qi and relax for a few minutes.

6. Spinning the Qi

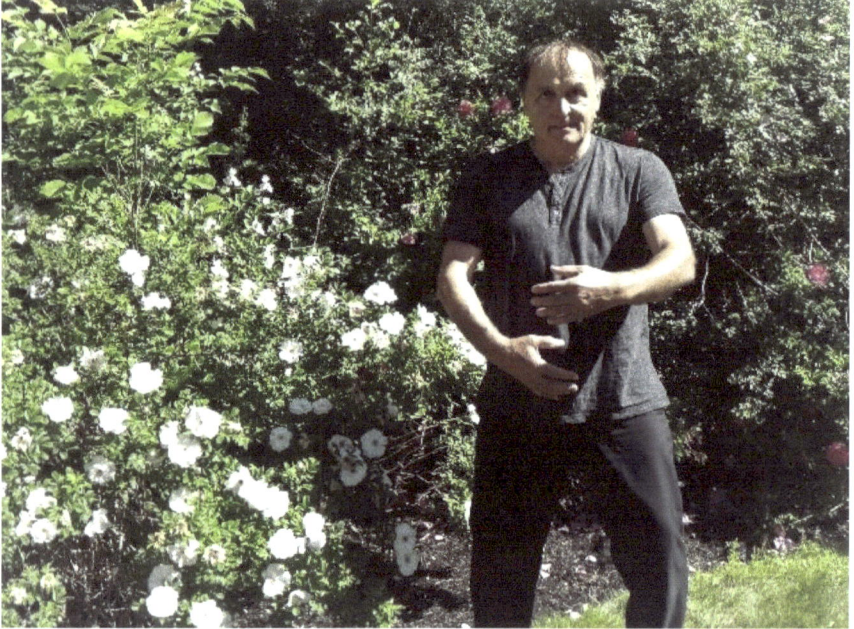

This method brings more Qi to the Lower Dantian strengthening both Yang and Jing Qi. The spinning of the Energy or Fire Ball strengthens the Belt Meridian which supports the circulation of Qi in the Conception Vessel helping prevent digestive, urinary and reproductive system problems.

Sit on the edge of a chair with palms facing down to conserve energy or stand with the arms hanging down along the sides of the body. Imagine there is a bright white ball of energy or a fire ball in the Lower Dantian.

Visualize the energy ball spin in the same direction as the Microcosmic Orbit, from the Qi Hai (Just below the navel) down to the Hui Yin (Center of pelvic floor) and around to the Ming Men (Mid lower back). Repeat until you feel heaviness or heat rise in the Lower Dantian.

Use the palms to intensify the spinning of the energy ball. With the palms facing the lower abdomen, one hand in front of the other, rotate the hands with increasing speed visualizing the energy ball turning in a circle in the same direction as the Microcosmic Orbit.

The movement of the hands is circular with the palms always facing the abdomen to develop a lot of Qi rotation. Breathe naturally. Rotate the hands 300 times. Continue by imagining the Qi ball turning in the lower abdomen from the Qi Hai, to the Hui Yin to the Ming Men. Place the Mind in the middle of the turning ball of energy.

Grow the size of the ball to include the Micro Cosmic Orbit, the whole body, the Earth, the Solar System, the Galaxy, and the Cosmos. Imagine that you are at the center of the energy ball which is rapidly rotating around you.

Then after a few minutes let the energy ball gradually get smaller and smaller. Maintain the spinning inside the Lower Dantian for a few minutes and even after the end of training.

When practicing in a group keep a comfortable distance from the other practitioners to reduce possible energy interference. When sensitivity to Qi increases you will become more aware of other people's energy patterns.

7. Smoothing the Qi

This exercise helps clear out dense Qi and re-establish energy flow and balance in the area between the hips and shoulders. It can be done sitting but it may be easier to do this exercise standing.

The palms hold an energy ball in front of the lower abdomen. Turn the left palm slightly upward and towards the body. Inhale, lifting the left hand to shoulder height. Exhale turning the palms slightly downward and return the palms to navel height. Repeat 6 times.

Immobilize the left hand and do the same movement with the right hand. Repeat 6 times. Then inhale lifting both palms to shoulder height. Exhale lowering both palms to navel height. Repeat 6 times. Focus the Mind on the area between the palms and the front of the body smoothing the wrinkles in the Qi fabric.

8. Turning the Water Wheel

This exercise builds Qi by favoring an exchange of energy with the Universe and the Tai Chi Pole located in the center core of the body.

With the palms facing each other, lower them to hip height then move them out and up the front of the body in a movement that resembles the turning of a water wheel.

Gather Qi as the arms move forward and out, move Qi down the center core of the body as the arms move inward and down, and release the Qi far into the earth as the hands reach the front of the hips. Repeat 10 to 30 times.

9. Joining Yin and Yang Energy Method

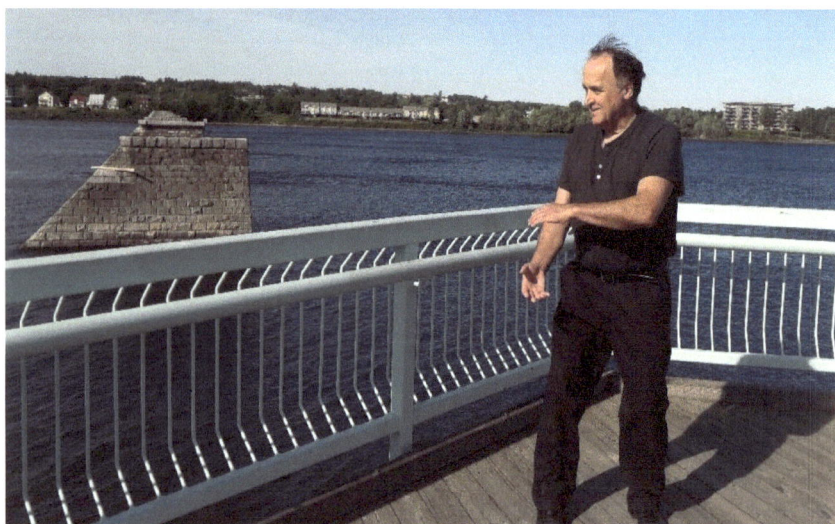

This exercise provides good palm energy to heal people.

In a standing posture, hold an energy ball in front of the Lower Dantian. Inhale Yang energy from the Universe into the lower Dantian via the Bai Hui or Crown Point. Exhale and relax. Let the energy come to the Lower Dantian. Repeat 6 to 9 times.

Then inhale Yin or Earth Energy in through the soles of the feet or Bubbling Spring Point, up the legs, and via the Hui Yin Point into the lower Dantian. Exhale and relax. Let the energy come to the Lower Dantian. Repeat 6 to 9 times.

Inhale Yang Qi from the Universe and Yin Qi from the Earth into the Lower Dantian. Exhale and relax. Let the energy come to the Lower Dantian. Repeat 6 to 9 times.

Stretch the Qi between the palms horizontally, vertically and diagonally letting the energy ball get bigger and bigger. Continue for a few minutes.

Then move the hips shifting the weight of the body from side to side. Continue stretching the energy between the palms. If your posture is correct the energy ball will stay in the palms and get larger. If your posture is not correct the energy ball will get smaller.

If this happens you need to correct your posture until the energy ball starts getting bigger once again. Practice for about 5 minutes. End by holding a Qi ball over the lower abdomen, palms about a fist-width away from the body. Rest the Mind in the Lower Dantian.

10. Humming Hands

Humming Hands open the six arm meridians and vibrate the Lao Gong Point (P8) located at the center of the palms. This exercise releases warm energy for healing.

In a standing posture with eyes open, raise the arms to chest height so they extend out to the front of the body, palms facing the earth as if resting on a large energy balloon. The fingers are slightly curled, and the arms are drawn back as the elbows drop slightly. On inhalation, open the palms and fingers wide as far as they will go comfortably. Relax on exhalation. Repeat stretching of the hands 6 to 12 times.

Inhale with Yin and Yang breathing into the Lower Dantian. (See breathing exercise in the **Joining Yin and Yang Energy Method**) The palms are rounded, arms and elbows relaxed. Exhale out the palms and the fingers, separating the fingers, and extending the palms forward.

Straighten the fingers and send the energy out. Simultaneously make the following sound to vibrate the palms. **HuuMmmmmm!**

Repeat 6 to 12 times. End by holding an energy ball in front of the Middle Dantian.

Caution: Don't create tension in the arms, shoulders, or back! If breathing becomes short while doing the exercise, the Kidneys may be weak, so you need to build more Kidney and Dantian energy. See Dan Gong or Lighting the Fire in the Lower Dantian exercise on page 51.

11. Playing with the Trees Method

The following is an excellent exercise to exchange energy with trees. Energy from trees helps reestablish the body's health. If you work around a tree, it helps slow the pulse rate, strengthens the immune system and makes you healthier.

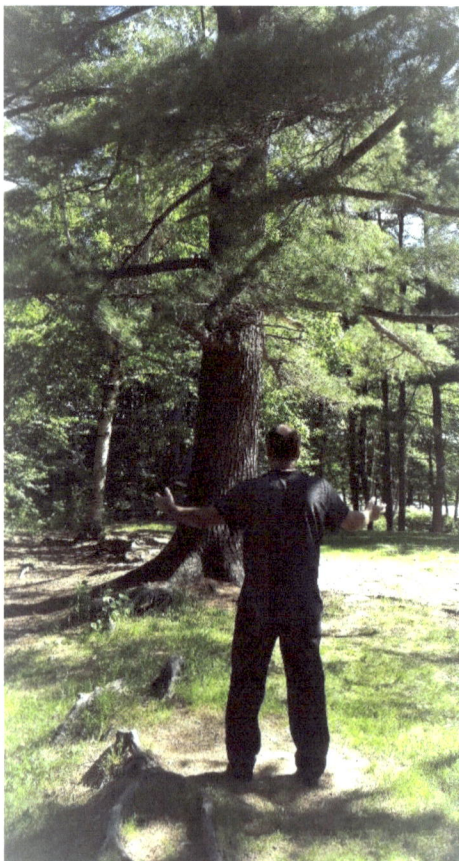

Every tree has roots and leaves. The roots are Yin energy from the earth. The leaves are Yang energy from the sky. Energy from the trees balances your energy making you feel good. In addition, with this exercise the inside of the nose can better defend against exterior pathogens.

Different trees have different energy. Most trees are good for the body, some are not. To cure specific health problems, you need to find the right tree. Different trees represent different colors which correspond to different organs. Cherry trees (Red) are good for the Heart, willow trees (Yellow) are good for the Spleen and

Stomach, while pine trees (Green) are good for the Liver. Always exchange energy with trees that are healthy.

Depending on the size of the tree, stand a minimum of 18 inches away from the tree in a relaxed posture. Smile from the Heart. The arms are open double shoulder width apart in front of the body, palms facing the tree. Open the three doors: Palm centers or Palace of Toil, Bai Hui or Crown Point and Hui Yin or Gate of Yin.

Practice Yin and Yang breathing. Inhale Qi and oxygen through the Hui Yin, Bai Hui and Lao Gong gates into the Lower Dantian. Gather energy through the doors. Exhale carbon dioxide and toxic Qi out the Hui Yin, Bai Hui and Lao Gong gates exchanging Qi with the tree. Practice for 5 to 10 minutes. When in a healthy environment you may substitute Yin and Yang Breathing with Pores or Whole-Body Breathing.

For the second part of this method, as you inhale, raise the arms with the palms facing up. As you exhale, bend the knees as the arms move down with the palms facing down. Inhale good energy through the three doors and exhale toxic energy out. Inhale, knees up, open doors. Exhale, bend knees, and clear out stagnant Qi. Smell the fragrance of the trees. Practice for 10 to 15 minutes.

At the end of the exercise inhale bringing the energy to the open mouth with the palms. As you exhale, swallow the saliva and energy down to the Lower Dantian. Repeat 3 to 6 times. Then place the palms over the lower abdomen and rest the Mind in the Lower Dantian.

It is better to do this exercise in the morning when the trees send out oxygen. With practice you will feel the palms become warm and tingly.

12. Sword Fingers

Sword Fingers is a high-level Qi Gong method as it opens the body's special functions. It gathers and builds cooling energy which can be used to treat infections and cool a patient's burn.

Stand feet wider than shoulder width apart, holding an energy ball in front of the lower abdomen. "Sit" on the feet. This saves energy and opens the Ming Men. Relax and correct the body - Bai Hui up, spine straight, Ming Men open, hips tuck in, chin in, nose in line with Lower Dantian. Open the Third Eye or Mid Eye Brow Point. Look far into the distance, into the big Universe.

Practice Reverse Belly Breathing throughout the form. Inhale Qi via the Crown Point down the center core of the body into the center of the abdomen. Exhale and let the Qi gather in the Lower Dantian. Repeat six to 12 times.

Inhale via the feet through the Hui Yin located at the center of the perineum into the lower Dantian. Exhale, letting the Qi gather in the lower abdomen. Repeat six to 12 times.

Inhale simultaneously via the Crown Point and pelvic floor or Hui Yin into the lower abdomen. Exhale letting the Qi gather in the lower abdomen. Repeat six to 12 times.

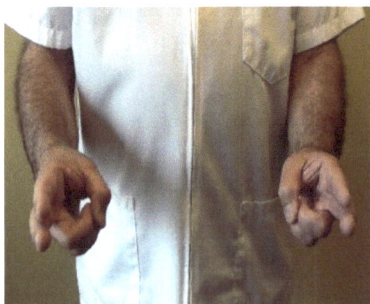

Adopt the sword finger posture with both hands, elbows parallel to the earth, fingers pointing forward. While moving 70% of the body weight to the front of the feet. inhale with reverse breathing simultaneously via the Crown Point and Hui Yin into the lower abdomen. While moving 70% of the body weight back to the heels, exhale out through the forearms, index and middle fingers far into the Universe. Repeat 6 to 12 times.

At completion, warm the hands by rubbing the palms together vigorously and massage the face and ears. Then holding the Yin Tang or the Mid Eyebrow Point with the left palm (Lao Gong), rub or massage Feng Qi or Wind Pool (GB 20), Feng Fu or Palace of Wind (GV 16) to Daz Hui or Big Vertebrae (GV 14). This rubbing/massage helps keep the cold out.

13. Emitting Qi in a Burst to Expel Toxic Qi

Stand relaxed and calm with feet parallel to each other, shoulder-width apart. Bend the knees slightly. Let the arms hang naturally to the side. Drop the tailbone down; suspend the crown of the head from above. Keep eyes open or half closed. Maintain natural breathing for 10 minutes with the tip of the tongue lightly pressed against the palate.

Then inhale through the nose, retracting the abdomen, focusing the Mind in the lower abdomen. Hold the breath while moving the respiratory diaphragm upward and downward a few times in a moderate to high speed to increase pressure in the abdominal cavity.

After a few repetitions, exhale through the mouth letting the abdomen extend outward to concentrate and emit Qi in a burst. This exercise can be used to destroy tumors and expel the toxic Qi via the breath and pores of the skin. Relax after each burst and elimination to help clear the Qi and Blood and resolve any cysts or tumors.

Repeat holding the breath and releasing bursts of Qi 6 to 9 times. Adjust the duration of holding of the breath to your individual condition. Increase repetitions as you become more comfortable with the exercise.

14. Shaking Method with Cleansing Breath

Everyone suffers from tired, stagnant or toxic Qi. The shaking method helps to dislodge toxic Qi and separate the good from the bad Qi.

Let the arms hang down to the sides of body. Bounce lightly, bending and extending the knees shaking the whole body. While shaking, relax each part of the body: Head; Shoulders; Neck, Arms, Forearms, and Hands, Chest; Abdomen; Hips; Groin, and Legs. Make sure every area of the body shakes. Practice the shaking method for 5 minutes. The body warms up if the exercise is done properly.

At the end of the method, visualize breathing in through crown of the head into the abdomen, and breathe stagnant Qi out the legs and feet deep into the earth. Bring Universal Qi from above the Bai Hui down the center core of the body, through the legs and feet, deep into the center of the earth. Repeat 6 to 9 times.

To end, bring the Mind to the center of the abdomen and rest for a moment. This will bring the Qi to the Lower Dantian and build energy. Feel the Qi growing. Keep and store energy in the Lower Dantian.

15. Closing with Self Massage with SOONG

The form ends with a massage of the abdomen, face and head. The abdominal massage helps consolidate the Qi in the lower abdomen and descend rebellious Qi helping resolve digestive issues, calming the Liver and the Spleen.

The facial massage beautifies the skin and releases tension in the neck and head area. The head massage strengthens the ears and Kidneys and helps open the Palace of Wind energy gate located at the back of the head just below the occipital protuberance.

- Standing heels almost touching, feet slightly turned outward, bring the palms to the navel. Men place right hand over left, women left hand over right.

- Massage the abdomen in a circular fashion 9 times in each direction. Increase the size of the rotations as you turn the palms in a counter clockwise direction. During this movement, the palms remain between the pubic bone and the sternum. Once you change directions, reduce the size of the rotations ending at the starting point over the navel.

- Raise the hands to the center of the chest and massage the centerline of the body with the heels of the hands down to the pubic bone. Repeat 9 to 18 times.

- Separate the palms and place them on the floating ribs. Massage down to the pubic bone. Repeat 9 to 18 times.

- Bring the hands to the front of the body, palms together. Rub the palms together vigorously until warm and place them over the front of the face, fingers pointing towards the sky.

- Massage the face by moving hands to the back of the head so the thumb and index fingers touch. Repeat 6 to 9 times.

- Rake the centerline of the head with the tips of the fingers 3 to 6 times.

- With the ears placed between the middle and index fingers, massage the sides of the ears by moving the hands up and down 50 to 100 times.

- Massage the ears by pressing the thumbs against the ears three times.

- With the thumb and sides of the index fingers, pull the ears out and then down.

- Pop the ears 3 times by placing the middle fingers in the ear opening, twisting the fingers twice in the same direction, and releasing.

- Drum the Qi by placing the cupped palms over the ears with the fingers lying on the back of the head. Drum 3 sets of 9 for each of the three following methods – alternating fingers, all fingers together, snapping middle finger over ring finger.

- Drop the palms to throat level, finger pads resting below the ears on the jaw line. In a twisting motion gently massage the sides of the throat with the base of the palms with alternating hands. Repeat 9 times. Repeat the same movement but with both hands 9 times.

- Bring the Qi down to the sides of the body with the palms and release the stagnant Qi deep into the earth. Gather Qi with the palms and place them over the abdomen, thumbs overlapping slightly at the navel, men right hand over left, and women left hand over right.

- Using the Mind, expand the body outward and inhale Universal Qi. Exhale with the sound SOONG vibrating the whole body. Repeat 3 to 6 times.

To end the form, you may choose to place the right fist in the left palm, look at your teacher and each student, and bow from the hips thankful for what you have learned.

Gathering, Moving and Balancing Qi

This style Of Qi Gong teaches Dan Gong or how to grow Qi in the Lower Dantian, as well as how to express its energy. Energy can only be used properly when you learn to gather and direct Qi with intent. When you are internally strong, externally you can do healing work.

In addition to Dan Gong, this form trains the practitioner to move Qi in the palms, in major acupoints, the Micro and Macro Cosmic Orbits, in the Shu and Mu Points, and in the 12 Regular Meridians.

1. Dan Gong or Lighting the Fire in the Lower Dantian

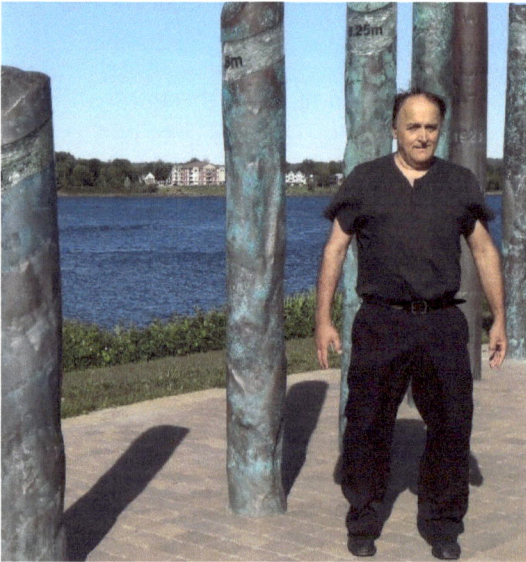

To light the fire in the Lower Dantian stand feet shoulder width apart, weight 70% on the Bubbling Spring or Kidney 1 Point, arms hanging loosely down the sides of the body. Inhale, contracting the abdomen and lifting the anus gently, moving the abdomen gently in and up. Exhale and relax, letting the abdomen expand naturally.

On inhalation, visualize the energy or Qi ball moving in a circular fashion from the navel to the Hui Yin to the Ming Men and back to the navel where you exhale and relax. Practice Reverse Belly Breathing for 5 to 10 minutes. Beginners start with only ten to 20 repetitions working their way up gradually to 100 repetitions.

This is a powerful exercise. It builds heat and Qi in the lower abdomen by massaging the internal organs. It creates a smaller space in the abdomen, moves the organs and creates more energy. If a space does not move it becomes stagnant and health problems can result. Movement creates energy.

In Daoism, the body is Yin and the eyes Yang. To bounce back the Yang, with eyelids closed or open, look into the Lower Dantian to light the fire and heat up the Yin. Feel you are there but not there. Do not think too much as it may lead to abdominal pain.

Use the eyesight to plant the Qi seed and let it grow naturally. Stay there but do not stare. Keep the Mind in the center of the Lower Dantian until the Kidneys feel heavy and warm. This means you are building original Qi. It may take two to three months to feel the heat in the Lower Dantian.

Sometimes you can feel the energy turning in a circle. If so put your Mind at the center of the circle. The Qi will automatically move to the Lower Dantian and circulate in the Micro Cosmic Orbit. First feel the energy in the Lower Dantian before circulating Qi in the Micro or Macro Cosmic orbits, otherwise nothing will be achieved.

A Mind that thinks too much will not circulate the Qi. Calm the Mind and relax the body.

This is a higher level of practice, like the way a baby breathes. It raises energy and makes you younger. Inhaling squeezes the internal organs up and exhaling lets them relax. This sponge process makes the organs more active, therefore there is more life. The body is weak when there is no activity. Tai chi is good external exercise, but by focusing on breath we exercise the internal organs.

Dan Gong increases sexual energy, helps avoid premature ejaculation and prolapse of the anus, uterus and Stomach. The lifting of the anus and perineum is good for the excretory system. It helps prevent hemorrhoids, colon cancer and localized infection. It can be combined with moving the Qi in the Micro Cosmic Orbit.

Once you feel the heat in the Lower Dantian guide it to the Bubbling Spring. Then your feet may feel warm. Do not let the Qi move beyond the feet or it will be lost.

2. Dropping the Heels to Release Qi

Standing with the weight of the body 70% on the heels, inhale with Reverse Belly Breathing letting the arms rise up to the front of the body shoulder height. The heels lift off the floor as the weight of the body moves to the front third of the feet. Exhale and drop the heels letting the arms fall to the sides of the body. Repeat 6 to 12 times.

The energy in the Lower Dantian may move down the legs to the Bubbling Spring and bounce back. Like a balloon, inflate the Qi outward and let it come back. The Qi moves to the feet and bounces back, relaxing the muscles and opening the joints and Crown Point. The person may look like they are flying.

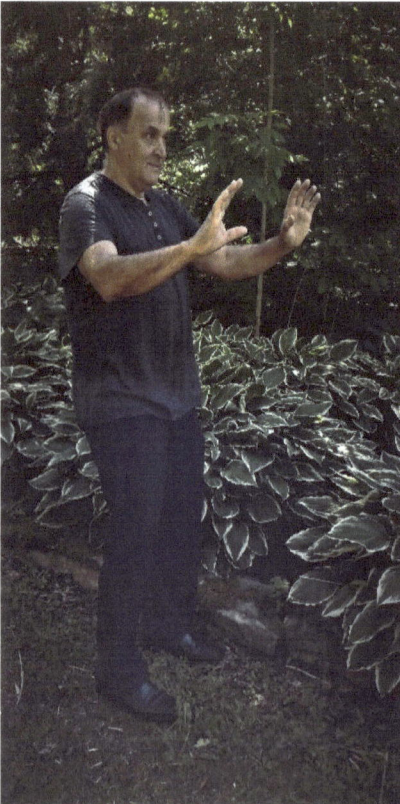

3. Gathering and Extending Qi - Front

Move the body weight to the front third of the feet. Inhale with Reverse Belly Breathing raising the arms to shoulder height in front of the body. Gather Qi by pulling the lightly cupped palms back towards the chest. As you exhale, abdomen expanding outward, extend the palms forward pushing the Qi through the palms towards the front of the body. Repeat 6 to 9 times.

4. Stretching and Compressing the Qi

Palms facing each other head width apart, on inhalation with Reverse Belly Breathing, expand the arms outward to shoulder width stretching the Qi. On exhalation, abdomen expanding, move the palms back to head width compressing the Qi. Repeat 6 to 9 times.

5. Gathering and Extending Qi - Sides

Inhale with Reverse Belly Breathing moving the arms to the sides of the body into a "T" formation, arms shoulder height, fingers pointing to the sky, palms extending out to the sides.

Exhale lowering the arms to hip height with the palms extending outward, knees slightly flexed.

As you inhale bring the pads of the fingers together raising the wrists and arms upwards back to shoulder height, straightening the knees. As you lower the arms on exhalation, lower the knees also dropping the tailbone down towards the earth.

The body weight shifts from front to back during the exercise, moving forward on inhalation and back on exhalation. Repeat 6 to 9 times.

6. Chakra Balancing

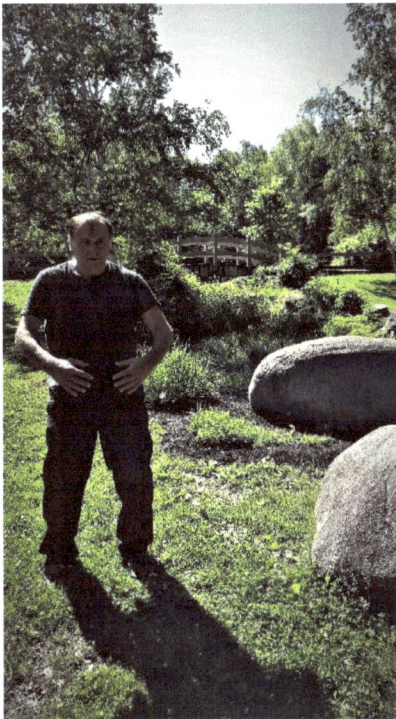

Stand, feet parallel, shoulder width apart, weight 70% on the heels. Inhale, opening the chest. Gather Qi with the palms and bring the Qi towards the front of the body "breast stroke fashion".

Exhale, rounding the back and extending Qi to the major energy centers or Chakras one at a time. Visualize sending the Qi through body to the corresponding Chakras centers at the back of the body, snaking the spine for each point in the following sequence.

- Reproductive Organs area to the tip of the Coccyx or GV 1
- Just below the navel to the Ming Men or GV 4
- Solar Plexus region to the center of the spine or GV 6
- Mid Chest Point to Spirit pathway or GV 11
- Base of throat to the Big Vertebrae or GV 14
- Mouth to the occipital protuberance at the Palace of Wind or GV 16
- Mid eyebrow point to the Jade Pillow or BL 9

Arch the back slightly and open the palms up and out to the sky, embracing the Universe, gathering Heaven's energy. Rise up on the toes. Feel the energy. Smile to the energy.

Straighten the back while coming back down onto the heels. Beam the energy with the palms down into the Crown Point. Lower the palms down the front of the body, guiding the Universal energy down the Ren or Conception Vessel to the Lower Dantian.

When the hands pass in front of the forehead, they adopt a prayer-hands position, moving down to the front of the Heart. Pivot the prayer hands while moving down to the abdomen, hands coming to rest in small triangle with the opening of the triangle over the Lower Dantian just below the navel. Rest the Mind in the center of the abdomen for a few moments. Repeat 3 to 6 times

7. Nine Gong Meditation (Nine Houses Meditation)

This Nine Gong or Nine Houses Meditation cleanses and energizes the three Dantians. This is a very ancient way of preventing disease, stopping toxic Qi from entering your body, and for preventing people from stealing your Qi. This is not a commonly known style of Qi Gong as it was traditionally practiced in China by people of high rank.

First become familiar with the following acupoints: Bai Hui (Hundred Meetings), Yin Tang (Hall of Impressions), Feng Fu (Palace of Wind), Shen Zhong (Chest Center), Daz Hui (Big Vertebrae), Qi Hai (Sea of Qi), Ming Men (Gate of Life), Hui Yin (Meeting of Yin), and Zhong Wan (Middle Cavity).

Imagine there is a small cylinder entering the body at the Crown Point or Bai Hui. Inhale universal energy through the cylinder into the center core of the body down to the Lower Dantian. Exhale stagnant Qi out the Crown Point far into the Universe. Repeat 3 to 6 times.

Imagine there is a small cylinder entering the forehead at the mid eyebrow or Yin Tang point. Inhale universal energy through the cylinder into the cranial cavity and exhale stagnant Qi out far into the Universe. Repeat 3 to 6 times.

Imagine there is a small cylinder entering the body at the Palace of Wind just below the nape of the neck. Inhale universal energy through the cylinder into the cranial cavity and exhale stagnant Qi out far into the Universe.

Imagine there is a small cylinder entering the Mid Chest Point into the chest cavity. Inhale universal energy through the cylinder into the chest cavity and exhale stagnant Qi out far into the Universe.

Imagine there is a small cylinder entering the Big Vertebrae into the chest cavity. Inhale universal energy through the cylinder into the chest and exhale stagnant Qi out far into the Universe.

Imagine there is a small cylinder entering the Sea of Qi Point located just below the navel into the abdominal cavity. Inhale universal energy through the cylinder into the abdomen and exhale stagnant Qi out far into the Universe.

Imagine there is a small cylinder entering the Ming Men point located on the lower back into the abdominal cavity. Inhale universal energy through the cylinder into the abdomen and exhale stagnant Qi out far into the Universe.

Imagine there is a small cylinder entering the Hui Yin point located at the center of the perineum into the center core of the body. Inhale universal energy through the cylinder into the caner core of the body and exhale stagnant Qi out far into the Universe.

Imagine there is a small cylinder entering the Solar Plexus or Middle Cavity providing access to all three cavities – cranial, chest and abdominal. Inhale universal energy through the cylinder into the three cavities and exhale stagnant Qi out far into the Universe. Rest for a moment with the Mind in the Lower Dantian.

Meditate on each house 3 to 6 times or do each of the houses once and repeat the whole sequence again until you feel the houses open and energized. Once you feel the Qi in the houses there is no need to continue the exercise.

8. Opening the Micro-Cosmic Orbit

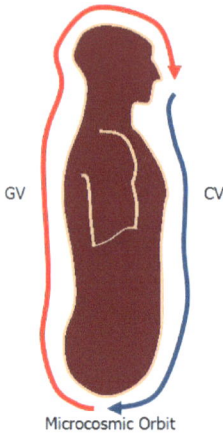

GV

CV

Microcosmic Orbit

Yin/Yang imbalance is the root of all problems. Maintain your own balance by performing the Micro-Cosmic Orbit which balances Qi in all Yin/Yang meridians. The Micro-Cosmic orbit is comprised of two special meridians, the Conception or Ren Vessel and the Governor or Du Vessel.

The Du Vessel primary pathway originates in the lower abdomen and emerges at the perineum. It passes through Du 1 or the Long Strong Point located between the tip of the coccyx and the anus. It runs up the spine to the nape of the neck. An interior branch enters the brain and ascends to the Bai Hui or Crown Point. The exterior branch moves along the midline of the head to the tip of the nose and upper lip, entering the mouth to end at Du 28, at the junction of the inner upper lip and the gum.

The Ren Vessel primary pathway arises at the center of the perineum between the reproductive organs and the anus. It ascends along the midline of the abdomen, chest, throat and jaw, terminating at Ren 24 between the chin and lower lip. An interior portion of the channel winds around the mouth connecting with the Du Vessel at Du 28.

There are ten activating points along the Micro-Cosmic orbit. First learn the location of these points.

1 - Qi Hai (Ren or CV 6 @ 1.5 cun below umbilicus pronounced Chi Hai)
2 – Hui Yin (Ren or CV 1 @ Center of Perineum)
3 – Chang Qiang (Du or GV 1 @ Tip of Coccyx pronounced Chang Chiang)
4 – Ming Men (Du or GV 4 @ L2)
5 – Shen Dao (Du or GV 11 just below T 5)
6 – Da Shui (Du or GV 14 – Just below C 7 Big Vertebrae pronounced Ta Choue)
7 – Feng Fu (Du or GV 16 @ below the occipital protuberance)

8 – Bai Hui (Du or GV 20 @ Crown of Head pronounced Bac Hui)
9 – Ying Tang (Mid Eyebrow Point)
10 – Dan Zhong (Ren or CV 17 @ Mid Chest pronounced Trang Song)

Two Types of Practice:
- Student does self-practice
- Teacher opens student's Micro-Cosmic Orbit

- Self Practice

Imagine a fireball. Send it via the Yin Tang or mid-eyebrow point down to the Lower Dantian. Feel the energy and warmth in the abdomen. Send the Mind to each of the acupoints along the Micro Cosmic Orbit. This opens the points and they may feel warmer. You can also chant the points if helpful. Then open the Micro Cosmic orbit and let the energy circulate faster and faster.

Activate the orbit three to ten times daily. Don't rush or force it. It is important to do it but not to overdo it. Too many times can burn you out.

The orbit can be experienced in many ways – feeling or seeing Qi. When your orbit is open, pictures and visions may come to you. Each person may have different experiences - memories, sounds, fragrances. This is normal. No worry!

Energy moves along various "stations" of the Microcosmic Orbit. If you are a feeling person and you don't feel a point, don't move to the next one until you feel the point as it isn't ready yet. This is especially true for the points at the Lower Dantian.

If you feel the whole orbit except for one point that is fine – continue practicing. Whether you feel the point or not, relax and continue to practice. You are still activating the orbit even if they are not sensing all nine points!

Finish with Open with the Universe Meditation ending with a face and ear massage. Rub the hands together activating the Heart and Pericardium meridians before massaging the face.

- Teacher Opens Student's Micro-Cosmic Orbit

To begin the student's eyes are closed with the tip of the tongue on the palate and the anus gently closed.

Both teacher and student imagine a fireball that enters the Yin Tang or mid-eyebrow point and descends into the Lower Dantian. Feel the energy and warmth in the Lower Dantian. Then both the teacher and student focus their Minds on the acupoints along the Micro Cosmic Orbit in the predetermined order listed above. The students Mind is with the teacher's Mind.

The teacher waits two to three minutes before chanting the orbit points. While pronouncing the names of each point out loud, the teacher sends Qi to these points. The Qi is moved from one point to the other opening all the ten points situated along the orbit.

The student does natural belly breathing through the entire exercise while the Mind focuses on the specific points the teacher will be chanting. Each orbit point is chanted 6 times. Once you feel the movement of the Qi in the orbit there is no need to continue the exercise.

To facilitate the training, the teacher can use sword fingers pointed at the 3rd eye, to pull the energy from there down to the Lower Dantian. Then the teacher lets the student circle the energy back around.

To finish practice Open with the Universe Meditation ending with a face and ear massage. Rub the hands together activating the Heart and Pericardium meridians and massage the face.

CAUTION:
Once the Qi is circulating in the orbit it is no longer necessary to continue practice.

Also, regarding breathing for the Microcosmic Orbit, normal breathing, asynchronous to the flow of Qi in Micro Cosmic Orbit is particularly safe. It can be dangerous to practice strong breathing when moving Qi in the orbit.

9. Opening the Macro-Cosmic Orbit

The Macro-Cosmic orbit is an extension of the Micro-Cosmic Orbit. It moves the Qi through the Regular Meridians located in the legs and arms. First focus on the Lower Dantian to build Qi. Take a few minutes to open the Micro-Cosmic orbit. Then bring the Mind back to the Lower Dantian for a moment.

Inhale, gathering Qi in the Lower Dantian. As you exhale use the Mind to move the Qi from the Lower Dantian up the center core of the body to the Middle Dantian or Chest Center. From here move the Qi outward to the armpits down the inside of both arms to the tips of the fingers, then up the outside of the arms and sides of the head to the Bai Hui, or Crown Point, located on the top of the head just above the ears.

At this point, let the Qi descend the center core of the body to the Lower Dantian where it spreads out to the outside of the hips and down the outside of the legs to the soles of the feet. From here the Qi moves up the inside of the legs to the groin and center of the Lower Dantian. Inhale gathering Qi in the Lower Dantian. Repeat 6 to 12 times or until you feel the Qi flowing in the orbit.

10. Balancing the Zhang Fu Organs (Yin/Yang) Organs

In Traditional Chinese Medicine the Shu-Mu Law groups certain acupuncture points together for the diagnosis and treatment of various disorders. These points are located on the front and back of the body and are called the Front-Mu or Alarm Points and the Back-Shu or Transporting Points.

Front Mu Points are located on the chest and abdomen near their respectively related Zang Fu organs. Each of the Zang Fu organs and the San Jiao has a corresponding Front Mu point.

The Back-Shu points are located on the back on either side of the vertebral column, near the spinal ganglia and their respective Zang Fu organs. Each of the Zang Fu organs has a Back-Shu point, as does the San Jiao.

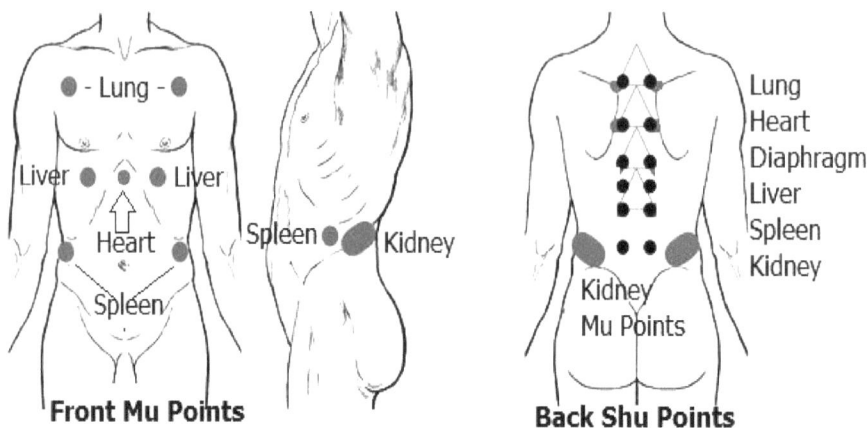

Front Mu Points

Lung - Lung

Liver — Liver

Heart

Spleen

Spleen — Kidney

Back Shu Points

Lung
Heart
Diaphragm
Liver
Spleen
Kidney

Kidney
Mu Points

Activating the corresponding Back Shu and Front Mu points regulates the balance between Yin and Yang. As each point alone has a strong influence on its corresponding organ, combining them boosts the effect of treatment. Clinical experience has shown that this combination usually has a better effect in full conditions when a sedating and soothing action is needed. It is used less in deficient conditions.

Traditionally, Back Shu points have often been prescribed for disorders of the Zang or Yin organs, while the Front Mu points have often been prescribed for disorders of the Fu or Yang organs. When using the Mind to balance the Yang organs, start with the front Mu Points. When balancing the Yin organs start with the back Shu Points.

For example, to balance the Lungs, a Yin organ, use the Mind to open the Yang Bladder 13 points located on the upper back. On inhalation breath into the points. On exhalation, follow the breath out of the points far into the distance. Repeat 3 to 6 times.

Then on inhalation follow the Qi through the Yin Lung 1 points located on the front of the body just below the shoulders. On exhalation, follow the breath out of the points far into the distance

The following chart provides the location of each Front Mu and Back Shu point for the Yin/Yang organs.

Organ	Back Shu Points	Front Mu Points	Position
Lungs	BL 13 @ T3	LU 1 - Slightly below lateral part of collar bone.	Same Level
Pericardium	BL 14 @ T4	Ren 17 - Chest center	Same Level
Heart	BL 15 @ T5	Ren 14 - Six inches above navel.	BL 15 is located slightly higher than Ren 14
Liver	BL 18 @T9	Liv 14 - Located directly below the nipples, in the 6th intercostal space.	Same level
Gall Bladder	BL 19 @ T10	GB 24 - Below nipples in the 7th intercostal space.	Same Level
Spleen	BL 20 @ T11	Liv 13 - Elbow height - lateral side of the abdomen, below the free end of the eleventh floating rib.	BL 20 is higher than Liv 13
Stomach	BL 21 @ T12	Ren 12 - 4 cun above navel	Same Level
Triple Warmer	BL 22 @ L1	Ren 5 - 2 cun down from the navel.	Ren 5 is slightly lower than BL 22
Kidneys	BL 23 @ L2	GB 25 - Located on the lateral side of the abdomen, on the lower border of the free end of the twelfth rib. Posterior to Liv 13.	Same Leve
Large Intestines	BL 25 @ L4	ST 25 - 2 cun lateral to the umbilicus.	Same Level
Small Intestines	BL 27 @ S1 – Level with bum crack	Ren 4 - Half way between the navel and the pubic bone.	Same Level
Bladder	BL 28 @ S2	Ren 3 - 1 cun above the pubic bone.	Same Level

To practice this form of Qi Gong focus on the organ systems that are out of balance or on the Yin organs uniquely following the Five Element Supporting Sequence: Lungs, Kidneys, Liver, Heart, and Spleen adding the Triple Warmer or San Jiao which is considered Yang but encompasses all three energy centers of the body.

Identify the location of the organs Mu and Shu points. Open the points with the Mind and follow the breath in and out of the points.

If you are treating a Yang Excess, start with the points on the Yin or front of the body. If you are treating a Yin Excess, start with the points on the Yang or back of the body. Meditate on each point for 3 to 6 breaths or until it feels open. Close by resting the Mind in the Lower Dantian for a few minutes.

11. Dragon Dancing in the Universe

This method clears out toxic Qi, gathers Universal energy, and energizes the body. The focus is on spontaneous movement and being one with the Universe. Widen the stance to twice the width of the hips.

The feet grow roots deep into the earth. Open the body with the Universe and let the Qi move you gently and naturally. Practice for five minutes or until the movement naturally comes to a stop. Finish by gathering Qi to the Lower Dantian.

Dancing and moving in a sea or universe of energy helps loosen all the body joints and sinuous tissue. The movement starts with the knees and shoulders, then arms and whole torso. You move in the big Universe, swim with the stars and heavenly bodies. Joy springs from the Heart! Let the movement be spontaneous! Be reassured that you are always in control and can stop the movement at any time.

Imagine the big sea, the Sun, the Moon, the solar system, the stars, and galaxies. Then towards the end, gather all the Qi into a ball. Circle it, play with it. Stretch the Qi between the palms. Finally, compress the Qi and place it in the Lower Dantian, and cover it with Diamond Hands.

12. Three Line Method to Relax the Body

In this method, we inhale through the Bai Hui or Crown Point down the center core of the body or Tai Chi Pole and exhale out down the outside of the body to the feet. This method is very relaxing. It harmonizes the Wei Qi or protective bio-energy field which radiates out from the body.

Stand in the Wu Ji posture, arms hanging down the sides of the body. Inhale universal energy into the Bai Hui or Crown Point of the head into the center of the body down to the Lower Dantian. Exhale Qi out the Bai Hui down the front of the body along the Conception Vessel and legs to the toes. Repeat 3 to 6 times.

Inhale universal energy into the Bai Hui or Crown Point of the head into the center of the body down to the Lower Dantian. Exhale Qi out the Bai Hui down the sides of the body to the feet. Repeat 3 to 6 times.

Inhale universal energy into the Bai Hui or Crown Point of the head into the center of the body down to the Lower Dantian. Exhale Qi out the Bai Hui down the back of the body along the Governor Vessel, and down the back of the legs to the heels. Repeat 3 to 6 times.

Inhale universal energy into the Bai Hui or Crown Point of the head into the center of the body down to the Lower Dantian. Exhale Qi out the Bai Hui down the front, sides and back of the body to the feet. Repeat 3 to 6 times.

13. Sky Sword with Macro and Micro 7 Stars

This form is very special as it gathers pure energy from distant regions of the Universe and integrates the energy into the practitioner's body. My first Qi Gong teacher, Master Weizhao Wu, explained that the purest Qi comes from the distant regions of the Universe.

Different kinds of Qi are required for different types of healing – general or special Qi. Healing Qi must be clear and pure. Sky Sword allows us to bring pure energy down from the Universe, refining our ability to gather higher-level Universal Qi.

When he taught me Sky Sword, Master Wu was not in favor of me sharing this form with others. Since his passing a few years ago, I have kept this form secret and only practiced it when there was no one present. The problem with keeping Sky Sword secret is that once I leave this earth the form may be lost to future generations.

Therefore, I decided to include Sky Sword and the accompanying Macro and Micro 7 Stars in this publication so others can discover its powerful Qi gathering and healing properties. Master Wu, who died a few years ago, had a big Heart. I am sure he will understand why I am sharing this information with you.

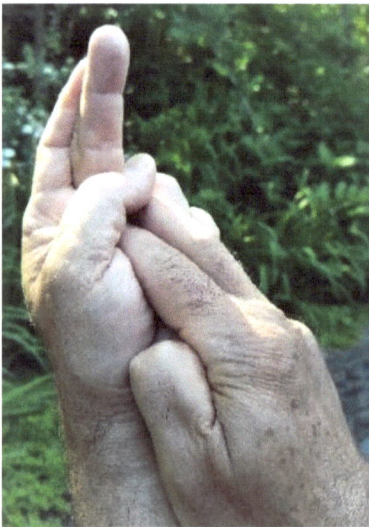

Objective: Direct Vital Qi from the Galaxy to Descend to your Head

Sitting or standing with a quiet Mind, adopt the Sword Hand as shown in the picture with the middle and index fingers pointing to the sky. Inhale. On exhalation raise the intertwined hands above the head. Inhale again gathering Qi from distant galaxies. On exhalation pronounce the sounds Yin Yien.

Inhale again gathering Qi from distant galaxies. On exhalation pronounce the following sounds: **Yin-He; Jing-Qi; Ju-Wo; Kuo-Lun** moving the hands down in a slight arc until the fingers point to the chin. At the end of the sequence the fingers continue to point to the sky and towards the chin.

Yin He (HA) = Galaxy
Jing Qi (CHI) = Essence
Ju Wo (WA) = Concentrate Mind
Kuo (KUIN) Lun = Name of Mountain symbolizing the head or Central Nervous System

Repeat the exercise a minimum of 12 times.

Seven Stars

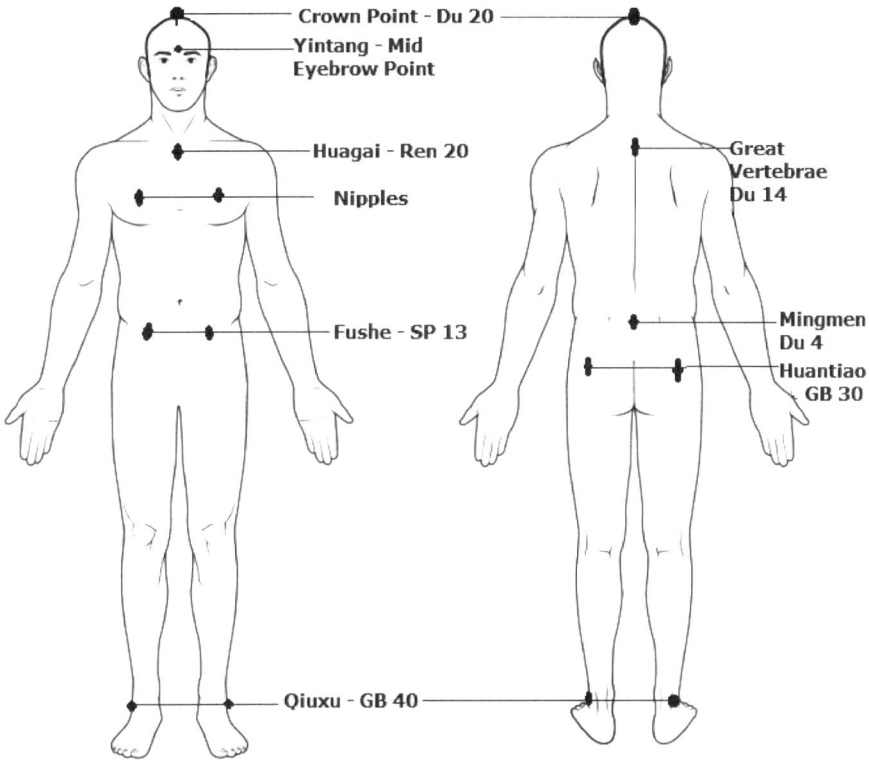

Crown Point - Du 20
Yintang - Mid Eyebrow Point
Huagai - Ren 20
Nipples
Fushe - SP 13
Qiuxu - GB 40
Great Vertebrae Du 14
Mingmen Du 4
Huantiao GB 30

Seven Stars allows you to integrate the Qi gathered from the Universe into the body via the Micro and Macro acupoints.

Micro 7 Stars Sequence:
- Crown Point (DU 20) =Top of the head above the ears.
- Big Vertebrae (DU 14) = First thoracic vertebrae.
- Mid Eyebrow Point (Yin Tang) = Between the eyebrows.
- Two Nipples
- Abode of the Fu (SP 13) = Inside hip bone about a fist-width away from the navel.

Macro 7 Stars Sequence:
- Crown Point (DU 20) =Top of the head above the ears.
- Magnificent Canopy (Ren 20) = Middle of chest in an indentation just below the sternal notch.
- Gate of Fire (DU 4) = On the midline of the lower back, in the depression under the spinous process of 2nd lumbar vertebra.

- Jumping Circle (GB 30) = Posterior to the hip joint.
- Mound of Ruins (GB 40) = In the ankle joint, in the depression anterior and inferior to the lateral malleolus.

Method to Place the Stars
Once you have practiced Sky Sword, place the energy in the Star Points starting with the Micro 7 Stars. Press each **Micro 7-Star** acupoint with the thumb and first two fingers for about 30 seconds. Apply lots of Qi to the pressure points. Repeat each set 3 to 6 times.

Then visualize the points filling with Universal Qi. In the beginning do one at a time. Then with practice group the points until you can do all of them at once. Continue until you feel the points opening and filling with Qi. Repeat the same exercise with the **Macro 7-Stars**. Finish by resting the Mind in the Lower Dantian.

14. Pores or Whole-Body Breathing

Visualize that all the pores of the body are open. As you inhale follow the breath moving in through the pores of the skin into the center of the abdomen. As you exhale follow the breath moving out of the pores of the skin far into the Universe. Practice for 10 to 20 minutes. Normally, 30 breaths equal approximately 5 minutes of practice.

15. Closing with Self Massage and SOONG (See previous Qi Healers Form)

Meditating on Acupuncture Points

This method of Qi Gong helps activate key acupuncture points located along various meridians or energy pathways. Each point has specific actions that balance various organ systems and physiological processes in the body.

Meditating on these points can reveal to the practitioner the true energetic nature of the points. In fact, it is believed that the ancient Chinese Qi Gong Masters discovered many of the functions of the various acupuncture points via this form of meditation.

The following points are a sample of some of the more dynamic points that can be activated through meditation. For each point, we detail their location and some of their major functions. After calming the Mind for a few minutes, focus on opening each point one at a time, following the breath in and out of the point.

Once you feel the energy in the point move on to the next location. It can be helpful to palpate the points first to determine their exact location.

Acu Point	Location	Function
Qi Hai – Sea of Qi	Ren 6 - Midline of body about three finger widths below the umbilicus.	Balances Yin & Yang. Strengthens the Lower Dantian & warms the Kidney Yang. Tonifies Jing & Yuan Qi. Good for the whole body & all organs.
Dan Zhong - Chest Center	Ren 17 - Midline of the body at center of the sternum midway between the nipples.	Tonifies Zhong Qi. Body's Qi centered here so important in regulating problems with Qi. Moves Qi in Heart & Lungs. Benefits the breasts & diaphragm. Treats cough & asthma.
Ming Men - Gate of Life	Du 4 - Midline of the lower back, in the depression under the spinous process of the 2nd lumbar vertebra.	Expels Cold. Nourishes Jing, Yuan & Yang Qi. Helps older men suffering from Yang Deficiency. Helps move Qi up the back. Treats lower back pain, weak knees & impotence. Focusing here for too long may generate too much Yang.

Hui Yin - Meeting of Yin	Ren 1 - Between the anus & the root of the scrotum in males & between the anus & posterior labial commissure in females.	Tonifies Jing & Yin Qi. Location of men's sperm & women's eggs. Combined with the Ming Men, it builds balanced energy. Can cultivate more Yin as Yin energy can be both Yin or Yang. Some older people suffer from Yin Deficiency.
Lao Gong - Palace of Toil	PC 8 - Palm center where the ring finger touches the palm of the hand.	Useful to scan energy, test the body as well as to gather & send out energy. Cools the Heart & Blood. Calms the Mind & the Stomach. If babies cry, touch this point & they will be quiet.
Yong Quan – Bubbling Spring	Kid 1 - On the sole of the feet, at a point 1/3 the distance from the base of the 2nd toe to the back of the heel.	Door to earth energy which is Yin. Floods the body with Kidney Yin. Roots the Body, Mind & Spirit. Lowers Qi. Clears Heat. Put the Mind there to help sleep. Treats headaches & High Blood Pressure. Nourishes Essence. Revives consciousness & rescues Yang.
Zu San Li – Leg Three Miles	St 36 - Under the knee, 4 finger widths to the knee cap & one finger width lateral to the anterior border of the tibia.	Vitality & longevity point. Raises Yang Qi. Clears Wind, Damp & Cold. Treats all Stomach & Spleen issues, & edema. Strengthens the immune system. Builds white Blood cells. Makes you stronger.
San Yin Jiao – Three Yin Intersection	SP 6 - On the medial side of the lower leg, 3 finger widths superior to the medial malleolus, in the depression close to the medial border of the tibia.	Builds Jing Qi. Nourishes Yin. Good for the Liver, Kidneys & Spleen. If you lose too much energy, use this point. Builds women's & men's sexual energy & energy for the Bladder. Regulates women's periods. Calms the Spirit, cools the Blood, & transforms Dampness. Treats depression.

Da Dunn – Great Sincerity	Liv 1 - On the dorsal aspect of the big toe, on its lateral side, proximal to the corner of the nail.	Clears out excessive Liver Yang. Clears the Mind. Calms the Shen. Treats eye issues, Liver headaches & heavy, painful periods. Makes Blood circulation go down more easily. Corrects body's energy.
Shao Shang – Lesser Shang	Lu 11 - On the inside of the thumb, proximal to the base of the nail.	Revives consciousness. Clears out Fire. Corrects burning in the Lungs, mouth, & teeth. Treats throat infection. Humidifies skin.

Moving Qi in the 12 Meridians

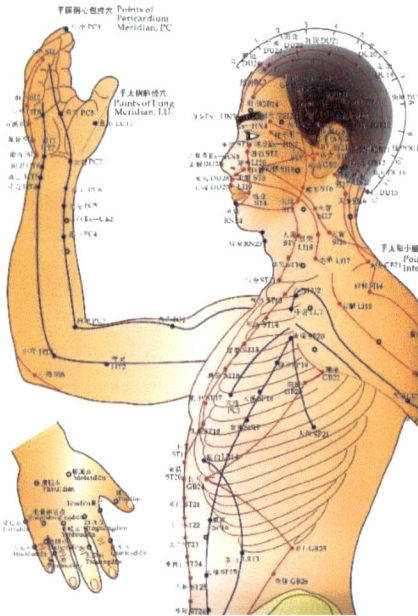

The human body has 12 regular meridians which flow away from or towards the center of the body. The Qi of the Yin meridians – Lungs, Heart, Liver, Kidneys, Spleen, Pericardium - flows away from the body while the Qi of the Yang meridians – Large Intestine, Small Intestine, Stomach, Bladder, Gallbladder, San Jiao or Triple Warmer– flows towards the center of the body. Each Yin Meridian is paired with a Yang Meridian – Lung/Large Intestine, Heart/Small Intestine, Liver/Gall Bladder, Kidney/Bladder, Spleen/Stomach, Pericardium/San Jiao. (See chart below)

Qi flows through all the 12 Regular Meridians in a 24-hour cycle. The energy of each organ meridian is strongest for two hours of each day. Keeping these channels open is very beneficial for good health.

This style takes time to master as it requires knowing the location of four acupuncture points situated along each of the 12 regular meridians. The points represent the first and last points on the meridian, plus the Yuan Source Point and He Sea Point.

The Yuan Sources points are the first to be activated for each meridian. These points are located at the wrists and ankles and are where the original or Jing Qi surfaces on the meridian. The He Sea points are located around the elbows and knees where Qi enters to a deeper level to communicate with the meridian's related organ.

Ming
Men

Qi
Hai

Hui Yin

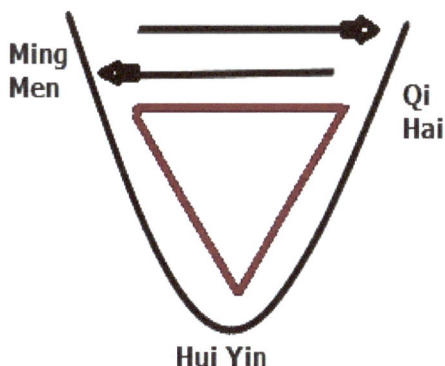

Before moving the Qi in the meridians, it is important to build strong Qi in the Lower Dantian. If the Qi in the lower abdomen is weak it will be very difficult, if not impossible, to move Qi on the meridians.

The following are two exercises that build strong Dantian energy. Practice these exercises before doing Meridian Qi Gong. They can be done in any position, sitting, standing or lying down.

Use the Mind to open the pathway between the Ming Men or Gate of Life and the Qi Hai or Sea of Qi. As you inhale follow the breath from the Ming Men to the Qi Hai. As you exhale follow the breath from the Qi Hai to the Ming Men. Repeat for 5 to 15 minutes or until you feel heat or heaviness in the Lower Dantian.

Another method to build strong Dantian energy is to open a circular pathway from the **Qi Hai to the Hui Yin to the Ming Men to the Qi Hai** and back in the opposite direction.

As you inhale follow the breath from the Qi Hai to the Hui Yin. Exhale to the Ming Men. Inhale to the Qi Hai. Exhale back to the Ming Men. Inhale to the Hui Yin. Exhale to the Qi Hai. Continue building the Qi for 5 to 15 minutes or until you feel warmth or heaviness in the Lower Dantian.

Once you have generated energy in the Lower Dantian focus on moving the Qi in the meridians starting with the Lungs. First use the Mind to open the Meridian and then move the Qi between the points: Yuan Source Point > He Sea Point > First Meridian Point > Last Meridian Point. This moves the Qi strongly in the meridian. Once Qi is flowing move to its paired meridian following the Meridian Energy Flow sequence.

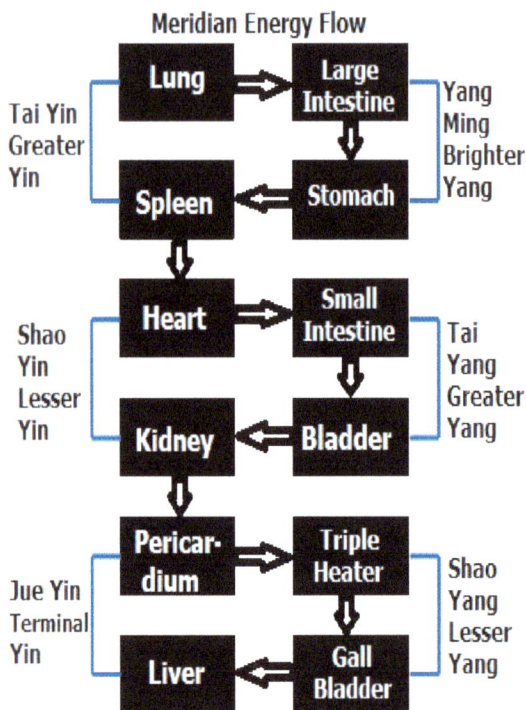

Meridian Energy Flow

1. Lung - Yin - 3 a.m. to 5 a.m.
Activation Points = LU 1 (Below Collar Bone); LU 5 (Elbow); LU 9 (Wrist); LU 11 (Outside Thumb)
Move Qi = LU 9 > LU 5 > LU 1 > LU 11

2. Large Intestine - Yang – 5 a.m. to 7 a.m.
Activation Points = LI 1 (Outside of index finger); LI 4 (Web of hand); LI 11 (External Elbow); LI 20 (Side of Nose)
Move Qi = LI 4 > LI 11 > LI 1 > LI 20

3. Stomach - Yang - 7 a.m. to 9 a.m.
Activation Points = ST 1 (Under Eyes); ST 36 (Outside of lower leg); ST 42 (Top of foot); ST 45 (Outside second toe)
Move Qi = ST 42 > ST 36 > ST 1 > ST 45

4. Spleen - Yin - 9 a.m. to 11 a.m.
Activation Points = SP 1 (Inside Big Toe); SP 3 (Above Big Toe Joint); SP 9 (Below Knee Inside of Leg); SP 21 (Zningeng)
Move Qi = SP 3 > SP 9 > SP 1 > SP 21

5. Heart - Yin - 11 a.m. to 1 p.m.
Activation Points = HT 1 (Armpit); HT 3 (Inside Elbow Fold); HT 7 (Inside Wrist Fold); HT 9 (End of Small Finger)
Move Qi = HT 7 > HT 3 > HT 1 > HT 9

6. Small Intestine - Yang - 1 p.m. to 3 p.m.
Activation Points = SI 1 (Small finger below nail); SI 4 (Knife hand after joint); SI 8 (Elbow); SI 19 (Front of ear lobe)
Move Qi = SI 4 > SI 8 > SI 1 > SI 19

7. Bladder - Yang - 3 p.m. to 5 p.m.
Activation Points = BL 1 (Inside of corner of eye); BL 40 (Behind Knee); BL 64 (Middle side of foot); BL 67 (Outside Little Toe)
Move Qi = BL 64 > BL 40 > BL 1 > BL 67

8. Kidney - Yin - 5 p.m. to 7 p.m.
Activation Points = Kid 1 (Bottom 1/3rd of feet down from toes); Kid 3 (Posterior to ankle); Kid 10 (Inside of knee joint); Kid 27 (End of color bone)
Move Qi = Kid 3 > Kid 10 > Kid 1 > Kid 27

9. Pericardium - Yin - 7 p.m. to 9 p.m.
Activation Points = PC 1 (Outside of Nipple); PC 3 (Elbow Fold); PC 7 (Wrist Fold); PC 9 (Outside of middle finger before nail)
Move Qi = PE 7 > PE 3 > PE 1 > PE 9

10. Triple Warmer - Yang - 9 p.m. to 11 p.m.
Activation Points = SJ 1 (Outside 4th finger below nail); SJ 4 (Back of wrist fold); SJ 10 (Elbow Tendon); SJ 23 (End of eyebrow around ear)
Move Qi = SJ 4 > SJ 10 > SJ 1 > SJ 23

11. Gall Bladder - Yang - 11 p.m. to 1 a.m.
Activation Points = GB 1 (Outside of corner of eye); GB 34 (Below outside of knee); GB 40 (Front of outside ankle); GB 44 (Outside corner of 4th toe)
Move Qi = GB 40 > GB 34 > GB 1 > GB 44

12. Liver - Yin - 1 a.m. to 3 a.m.
Activation Points = Liv 1 (Outside big toe); Liv 3 (Depression between small and big toe); Liv 8 (Inside Knee); Liv 14 (Below rib)
Move Qi = Liv 3 > Liv 8 > Liv 1 > Liv 14

Once you are good at moving the Qi in the 12 Regular Meridians the energy will move in the whole network by opening the first (Lung 1) and last (Liver 14) points. After moving the Qi on all the meridians rest the Mind in the Lower Dantian for a few moments to consolidate the Qi.

Five Element Qi Gong

According to Traditional Chinese Medicine there are six paired organ systems and regular meridians in the body. Six organs are considered Zang or Yin organs and six are considered Fu or Yang organs. They are the:

Yin Organs	Yang Organs
Kidney	Bladder
Heart	Small Intestines
Lung	Large Intestines
Liver	Gallbladder
Spleen	Stomach
Pericardium	Triple Warmer or San Jiao

These organ systems are paired by their function. The Triple Warmer is not an organ but represents three distinct regions of the body responsible for the management of fluids and the transformation of energy or Qi. The Pericardium is not an organ but the covering of the Heart. It acts as the Heart's protector.

Each organ has a corresponding meridian system like the branches of a tree that reach out to various parts of the body. During a 24-hour period the energy of the body circulates through all twelve organ systems via their meridians in a predetermined pattern.

Any blockages in the meridian network will eventually affect the related organ system. Also, imbalances in the organs will eventually affect the flow of Qi in the related meridian network.

Each organ vibrates at a unique energy frequency generating a specific sound and color. Over the years the sounds have been interpreted differently by various Qi Gong Masters. The understanding of the exact sounds may have been complicated by their translation from Chinese to English.

I have adopted the sounds that are commonly used by well-known Qi Gong Masters. I have chosen the sounds that I feel are the most effective in releasing stagnant Qi in the targeted organ systems. Intent and focus are important when practicing the healing sounds and Qi Gong.

Organ System	Organ Color	Organ Sound
Kidneys	Dark Blue or Black	**Chwa...a...a...y**
Heart	Red	**Haw..w..w..w**
Liver	Pearl Green	**Shu...e...e...e**
Lungs	White	**See...e...e**
Spleen	Yellow	**Huu...u...u**
Triple Warmer	Orange Red	**Shee...e...e**

For more information on the Healing Sounds refer to my first book on Qi Gong entitled The Power of Qi for Health and Longevity under the heading Healing Sounds.

The Five Element Qi Gong style combines the healing sounds, organ colors and specific body movement to help strengthen each organ system. I have divided the style into smaller segments to facilitate the integration of its movements and visualizations.

Method 1: The first method uses a ball of fire to warm up the targeted organ and intensify its natural color. Sit comfortably on the edge of a chair. Once you achieve a state of inner quiet, imagine a ball of fire hovering at the mid-eyebrow point or Yin Tang.

After a few moments, let the ball of fire enter the Yin Tang and move to the pineal gland located at the center of the head. Then let the fireball drop to the targeted organ.

As the organ warms up it creates more energy and more color. For example, imagine the ball of fire entering the Yin Tang, moving to the pineal gland, and dropping down to the Heart. As the Heart gets warmer, its Red color intensifies. Hold this visualization for a few moments before moving to another organ.

Method 2: Another method combines the color of the organ with its healing sound. Once you achieve a state of inner quiet, inhale while focusing on the healthy and vibrant color of the targeted organ.

Exhale pronouncing the organ's healing sound vibrating both the targeted organ and its opening to the exterior. After completing the sequence rest the Mind in the Lower Dantian for a few moments or until the area gets heavy or warm.

Organ System	Exterior Opening
Kidneys	Ears
Heart / Triple Warmer	Tongue
Lungs	Nose
Liver	Eyes
Spleen	Mouth

Method 3: The final version of this Qi Gong style adds body movement to the mix as well as the movement of Qi in the related meridian network. The Triple Warmer, although considered to be a Yang Organ, is included in this method due to its important role in managing Qi and fluids in the body.

First adopt a standing posture, with the arms hanging to the sides of the body, weight 70% on the heels. Practice Open with the Universe Meditation with the healing sound SOONG. Using the Mind, expand the body outward as big as the Universe. Inhale with Relaxed Abdominal Breathing gathering Universal Qi. Exhale pronouncing the healing sound SOONG, vibrating both the nose and the whole body. Repeat 10 to 30 times.

Following the controlling cycle of the Five Element Theory (See page 99), practice the Colors, Sounds and Body Movement for each of the five major organ systems (Kidneys, Heart, Lungs, Liver, Spleen) followed by the Triple Warmer. The sequence of movements for each organ system may vary slightly.

First inhale focusing on the vibrant and healthy color of the target organ while simultaneously initiating the specific body movement to compress the organ and open its meridian.

On exhalation, complete the body movement, pronouncing the healing sound which vibrates the organ and the exterior opening for that specific organ system. Using the Mind, follow the movement of the Qi in the organ's meridian or energy pathway. Exhalation is longer than inhalation.

Before moving to the next organ system, rest the Mind in the Lower Dantian for a few moments or until the area gets heavy or warm.

Kidneys

This style moves the energy in the Kidney organ system. It is comprised of two movements: Looking Behind to Cure Disease and Injury or Spinal Twist, and Kidney Qi Gong.

Standing with feet shoulder width apart, hold an energy ball with the palms facing the lower abdomen. After a few minutes turn the hips to the side 45 degrees, with the back leg soft but straight, and front leg bent so the knee tracks over the center of the front foot.

Rotate the spine to the closed side looking at the back heel. Move the front hand to the front of the forehead, about one fist-width away, and the back hand to the front of the lower back, about one fist-width away. Hold the posture and breathe 6 to 9 times.

Return to center, with the palms holding an energy ball in front of the lower abdomen. Rest the Mind in the Lower Abdomen for a few minutes or until it feels heavy or warm. Repeat the Spinal Twist on the opposite side. Hold the posture and breathe 6 to 9 times before returning to center. See second photo on page 89.

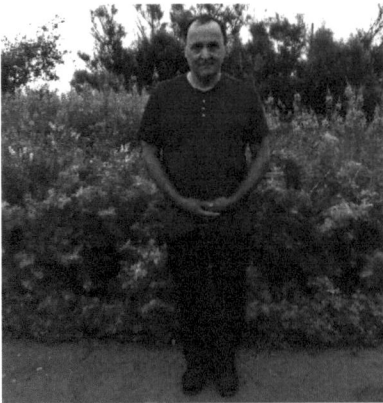

Place the palms over the Lower Abdomen just below the navel, left hand first for men and right hand first for women. Shorten the stance so that the heels are touching. Move 70% of the weight of the body to the balls of the feet.

After resting the Mind in the Lower Abdomen for a few minutes, place the tip of the tongue gently on the upper palate as far back in the mouth as you can comfortably like a sail pointing to the roof of the mouth. Inhale gently contracting the abdomen and lifting the anus, visualizing the vibrant Midnight Blue color of the Kidneys.

On exhalation, release the abdomen, pronouncing the healing sound **Chwa...a...a...y.** While exhaling, vibrate both the Kidneys and the ears, following the movement of Qi along the Kidney meridian, from the center of the feet up the inside of the legs to the groin, ending at the medial end of the collar bone. Repeat 9 to 12 times. End this sequence by resting the Mind in the Lower Abdomen for a few minutes or until it feels heavy or warm.

Heart

This style moves the energy in the Heart organ system. Feet shoulder-width apart, move the body weight to the heels, with the palms holding an energy ball in front of the Lower Abdomen.

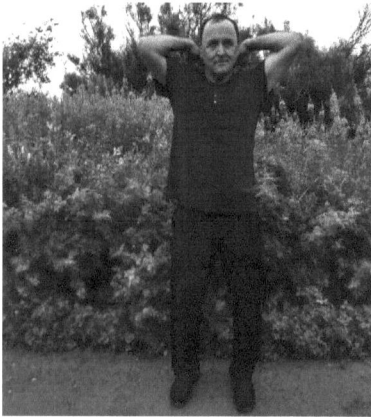

On inhalation, imagine the vibrant Red color of the Heart while you raise the arms up the front of the body, moving the palms behind the head with elbows facing upward. There is a feeling of openness in the Heart region. The fingers reach towards the first thoracic vertebrae or Du 14. Extend the elbows upward to help stretch and open the Heart meridian which flows from the armpit down the inside of the arm and forearm to the little finger.

With the mouth wide open, and the tip of the tongue gently placed on the inside of the lower teeth, exhale with the healing sound **Haw...w...w...w** vibrating the Heart and tongue, while following the movement of Qi along the meridian.

Simultaneously lower the palms to navel height to a holding-an-energy-ball posture. Rest the Mind in the center of the abdomen for a few moments or until it feels heavy or warm. Repeat the exercise 9 to 12 times.

Lungs

This style moves the energy in the Lung organ system. Lift the arms to shoulder height forming a "T". On inhalation expand the chest outward. Visualize clear, fresh vibrant white Lungs.

Rotate the forearms outward to open the Lung meridian which runs from the front sides of the chest near the armpits down the inside of the arms and forearms, to the inside of the thumbs.

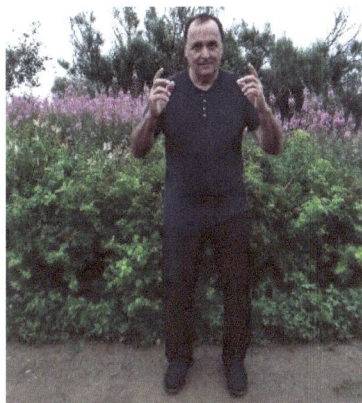

As you exhale, with the mouth slightly open and the tip of the tongue lightly pressed against the lower teeth, pronounce the healing sound **See...e...e...e** vibrating the Lungs and the nose.

The arms move to the front of the body, hands in a lightly closed fist. Imagine you are squeezing the Lungs like a sponge to expel water. Visualize stagnant energy moving out of the Heart and Lungs. Repeat 9 to 12 times before resting the Mind in the Lower Abdomen.

Liver

This style moves the energy in the Liver organ system. Feet are shoulder-width apart in a Standing-on-Posts posture. While holding an energy ball in front of the lower Dantian, rest the Mind in the middle of the abdomen for a few moments. Then inhale visualizing the vibrant Green color of the Liver.

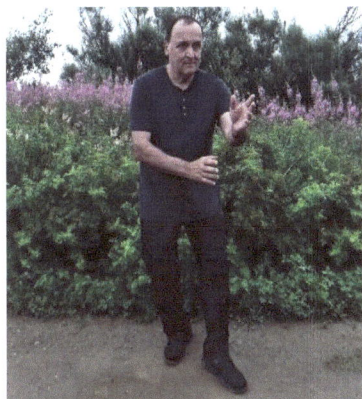

As you exhale rotate the hips to face diagonally into a defensive "T" stance shifting the weight of the body forward straightening the back leg and bending the front knee, so it tracks over the center of the front foot. Keep both knees soft. Extend the palms outward as if holding a sword. Pronounce the healing sound **Shu...e...e**.

Smile with the center of the lips lightly touching. The tongue is cupped and with the tip loosely placed on the inside of the upper teeth. The sound moves out the corner of the lips vibrating the sides of the mouth.

Imagine Qi moving up the Liver meridian which moves up the lateral side of the big toes to the inside of the legs and groin, up to the floating ribs, moving internally up to the sides of the mouth, behind the eyes to the Crown point on the top of the head.

The Liver opens to the eyes. Therefore, during this exercise intentionally open the eyes wide on exhalation to positively affect the Liver.

On inhalation, the body moves back slightly so the weight is 70% on the back leg. Let the Qi drop from the top of the head down to the mouth. At this point the front heel is slightly raised, with the weight of the front leg resting on the ball of the front foot. The front leg is empty, the back leg is full.

Inhale visualizing the vibrant Green color of the Liver. As you exhale extend the body forward with the palms in a defensive stance, once again pronouncing the healing sound **Shu...e...e...e** with the eyes wide open looking far into the distance. Let the healing sound vibrate the Liver, and the sides of the mouth. Follow the Qi up the Liver channel to the Crown of the head.

Inhale, moving the body weight to the back leg. Let the Qi drop down to the mouth from the Crown point. Repeat 6 to 9 times before returning to the holding-the-energy-ball posture. Repeat the same exercise on the opposite side.

Spleen

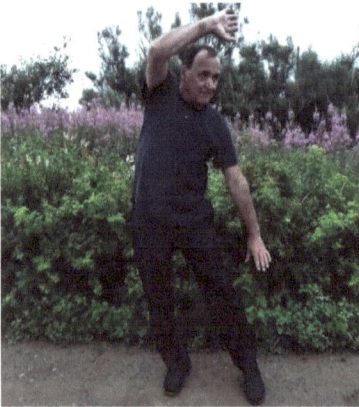

This style moves the energy in the Spleen organ system. Place the hands at the front of the body as if holding a ball encompassing the area from the navel to the bottom end of the sternum.

Palms facing each other, hold an energy ball with one hand on top and the other underneath. Turn the ball in a circle ending with the left hand on top. Inhale focusing the Mind on the Spleen. Imagine its deep Yellow color while moving 70 percent of the body weight to the right leg.

Exhale, extending the left palm down the side of the left leg, and the right palm upwards towards the sky. Raise the left heel off the ground moving the hips laterally towards the supporting leg to help open the Spleen meridian which moves from inside the big toes up the inside of both feet and legs to the groin. From here the Qi moves to the outside of the ribs to below the collar bone and down to a point four finger widths below the armpit.

Look in the general direction of the raised heel. While exhaling, pronounce the Spleen healing sound **Huu...u...u.** To pronounce the sound, the lips are rounded, the jaw is slightly open, and the tongue curled slightly downward. The Spleen and the inside of the mouth vibrate while pronouncing the sound.

Inhale, dropping the left heel, moving the body back to center, arms to a "T" stance and then into the holding-the-energy-ball posture. Rotate the energy ball a few times ending with the right hand on top. Repeat the same movement on the opposite site. Repeat again on both sides 9 to 12 times.

Triple Warmer

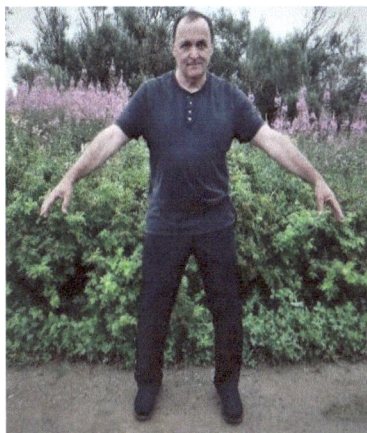

The Triple Warmer is also known by its Chinese name, San Jiao. It has no equivalent in modern Western Medicine. One traditional description of the Triple Warmer is the "Official in Charge of Irrigation".

The Triple Warmer extends from the base of the tongue to the pelvic floor. The Lower Warmer is in the pelvic region, at the level of the hips. The Middle Warmer is in the abdomen, at the level of the floating ribs, and the Upper Warmer is in the thorax region, at the level of the shoulders.

The Triple Warmer Meridian moves from the outside of the ring finger up the outside of the hand, forearm and arm, to the Great Vertebrae (First Thoracic Vertebrae or T1) around the back of the ear to the outside of the eyebrow. The Triple Warmer is a Yang Organ.

The Triple Warmer distributes the energy that is taken from the air we breathe, the food we eat, and the water we drink to different parts of the body.

To cleanse the Triple Warmer, stand feet shoulder width apart, with the arms resting along the sides of the body. Bend the knees slightly while breathing into the **hip area**. At the same time, lift the arms from the sides of the body approximately two fist widths imagining the vibrant Orange Red color of the Lower Warmer.

Exhale straightening the knees while moving the palms back to their original position. On exhalation pronounce the healing sound **She...e...e** vibrating the Lower Warmer and the tongue. The mouth is slightly open with the tip of the tongue gently placed on the lower teeth. Observe the Qi move in the Triple Warmer Meridian. Repeat 6 to 9 times.

While flexing the knees, breathe into the **floating ribs**. At the same time, let the palms move away from the sides of the body approximately four fist widths. Imagine the vibrant Orange Red color of the Middle Warmer.

Exhale straightening the knees slightly while lowering the palms to their original position. As you exhale pronounce the healing sound **She...e...e** vibrating the Middle Warmer and the tongue. The mouth is slightly open with the tip of the tongue gently placed on the lower teeth. Observe the Qi move in the Triple Warmer Meridian. Repeat 6 to 9 times.

Finally, bend the knees while breathing into the **shoulder area**. At the same time, raise the arms from the sides of the body approximately six fist widths. Imagine the vibrant Orange Red color of the Upper Warmer.

As you exhale pronounce the healing sound **She...e...e** vibrating the Upper Warmer and tongue. The mouth is slightly open with the tip of the tongue gently placed on the lower teeth. Observe the Qi move in the Triple Warmer Meridian. Repeat 6 to 9 times.

With the palms facing each other, head-width apart as if holding an energy ball, inhale raising the arms shoulder height to the front of the body. Rotate the forearms so the thumbs point down towards the earth. Open the arms wide into a "T".

Exhale lowering the hands until the thumbs rest on the sacrum palms together, opening the chest. Inhale, imagining the Orange Red color of the Triple Warmer. Then exhale moving the arms back to the holding-the-energy-ball frontal position while pronouncing the healing sound **She...e...e** and observing the Qi move in the Triple Warmer meridian. Repeat 6 to 9 times.

Closing: Relaxation with Soong

The word SOONG means relaxation of the Mind, Spirit and Body. It implies quietness, softness, flexibility, sinking, openness and emptiness as well as being free of obstructions.

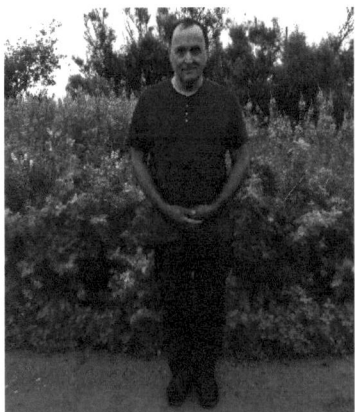

In the standing posture, inside of the heels lightly touching, place the palms over the Lower Dantian, right hand over left for men and left hand over right for women. Relax for a moment with the Mind in the center of the abdomen as shown in the picture.

Then inhale using the Mind to open the body as big as the Universe. When you exhale, pronounce the healing sound SOONG. When pronouncing the word SOONG, let the nose and body vibrate with the healing sound.

Relax the whole body from head to toes 6 to 9 times.

Dragon Dance 17-Style Form

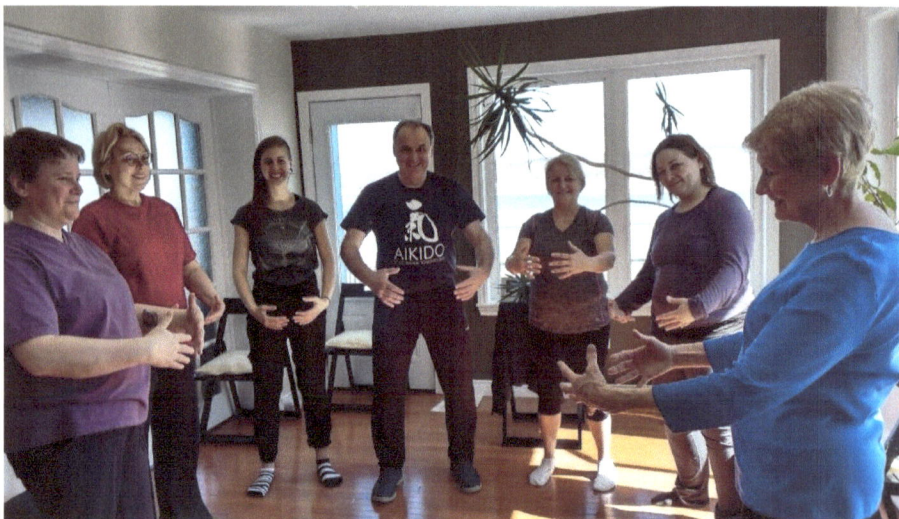

In China when people go to the local park to practice Qi Gong they often say that they are going out to play. While playing we are relaxed, happy, and spontaneous. This is the true nature of Qi Gong.

It is easy to get caught up in the technical aspects of Qi Gong memorizing forms created by one's teacher or one of the many Qi Gong forms found on the internet. Once we become familiar with a method of practice we sometimes find it difficult to see the value of other styles.

I have always found pleasure in discovering new forms of Qi Gong. Each practice session brings a new mix of techniques that expresses how I feel that day. Once the Qi Gong seed is planted, it will sprout and grow into a unique expression that respects each person's needs, experiences and abilities.

My first Qi Gong teacher, Weizhao Wu, would say that each day brings new energy. Our planet is continually moving in a Galaxy and Universe that are also in constant motion.

The Universal energy that envelopes us is never the same. Also, our internal energy changes minute by minute influenced by our emotions and the surrounding environment.

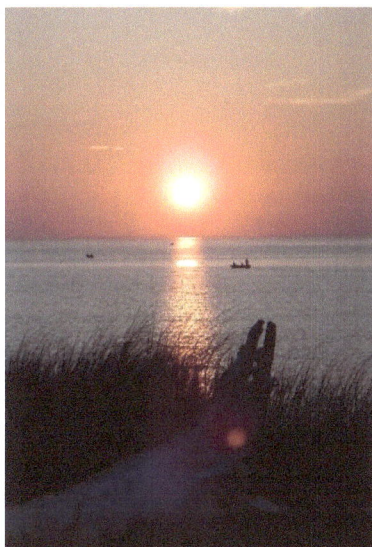

Therefore, it is good to learn to adapt to our personal needs and to the place where we find ourselves in the Universe at any given time. To help develop this ability, we often start a Qi Gong practice with Open with the Universe Meditation or Relaxed Abdominal Breathing.

This helps us connect to our inner self, to let go of ingrained tension, and to blend with the Universal energy present that day. Within this context, I felt it fitting to add to my third book on Qi Gong a style that represents the various aspects of my training in Qi Gong, Aikido, Yoga and Tai Chi.

The form, which starts with the Eight Diaphragm Breathing Method, incorporates exercises of stillness, movement and form born of the Martial and Healing Arts.

The Dragon Dance 17-Style Form lends itself to both Relaxed Abdominal Breathing and Reverse Abdominal Breathing. The recommended breathing method will be indicated for each style that makes up the form. Choose the breathing method that best suits your needs.

Let's play.

1. Eight Diaphragm Breathing

After relaxing in a standing posture with Relaxed Abdominal Breathing for up to 5 minutes, practice the Eight Diaphragm Breathing Method as described earlier in this book on page 37 under the Qi Healers 15-Style Form.

After moving the Eight Diaphragms 6 to 12 times, focus on opening every cell in the body on inhalation, and relaxing every cell in the body on exhalation. Imagine the cells are opening and closing like the movement of a Jellyfish swimming in the ocean.

Repeat 6 to 12 times before moving to the next exercise.

2. Raise the Arms to Collect Qi

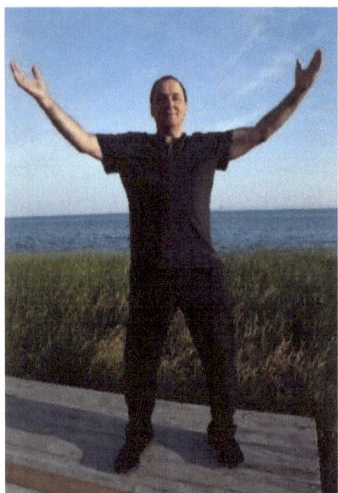

On inhalation, with Relaxed Abdominal Breathing, turn the palms outward while raising the arms up the sides of the body until the palms are facing the top of the head. On exhalation, lower the arms to the front of the body turning the palms at shoulder height so they face forward as if holding a ball. Continue lowering the arms to the height of the lower abdomen turning the palms so they face the body. Hold the Qi in the lower abdomen for a few moments before repeating 6 to 9 times.

3. Drop the Arm Back, Push the Palm Forward

Blending with the movement of the previous style, pause the arms at shoulder height with the palms facing away from the body. Look through the space between the palms far towards the horizon.

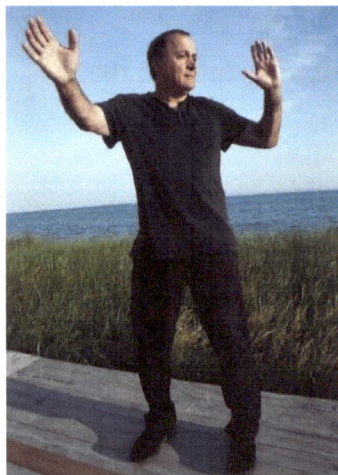

After a few moments, on inhalation with Relaxed Abdominal Breathing, drop the left arm down and to the side of the body, letting is swing back into a side facing "T" stance.

Look towards the back hand. Turn the back palm so it faces towards the front and, on exhalation, push the palm forward following it with the eyes returning to the starting posture, as shown in the picture. Look between the palms far into the distance. Repeat the same movement on the opposite side. Do left and right 6 to 9 times.

Once you are comfortable with the movement, try practicing reverse Belly Breathing during this style.

4. Palm Strike with Angry Eyes

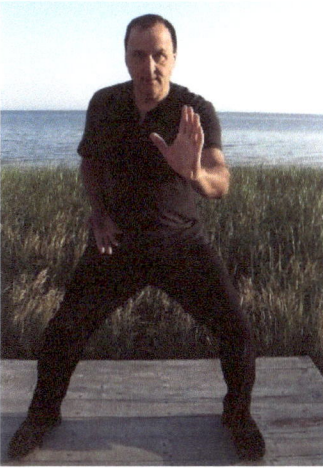

Rotate the forearms so the palms face up and place the back of the hands on the hips. Open the feet wide into a deep horse stance. Drop the tail bone down to straighten the lower back.

Exhale while extending the left palm forward into a palm strike. Open eyes wide. Inhale moving the right palm forward while retreating the left palm. Both hands meet in front of the abdomen. When both hands meet, rotate the palms so the right hand is on top.

Exhale while extending the right palm forward into a palm strike. As the right palm moves forward, the left palm moves back to the resting position on the outside of the hips palm facing up. Repeat on the opposite side. Do 6 to 9 repetitions.

When the palms meet in front of the body the Qi ball is turned 180 degrees. On extension of the palm, pronounce the sound **YYYAAAHHH** with angry eyes. Practice Relaxed or Reverse Belly Breathing.

5. Single Whip with Push Down

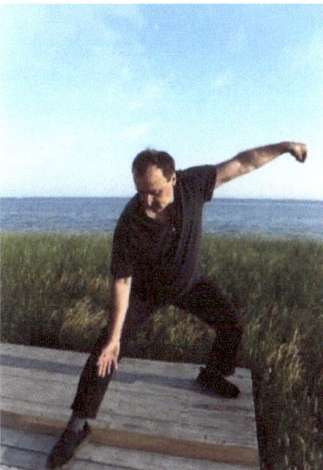

With the right palm extended forward into the palm strike, inhale releasing the left palm from the hip moving to the side of the body into a Single Whip with the pads of fingers touching and the back of the wrist extending up towards the sky.

Drop the hips, bending the left leg ensuring the knee tracks above the center of the left foot. Move the right palm down the inside of the extended right leg. Exhale, turning the hips so they face towards the front leg rotating the back forearm at the same time, so the fingers point towards the sky. Move the hips forward bending the front leg and straightening the back leg. Keep the knees soft. During this style practice Relaxed or Reverse Belly Breathing.

6. Standing on One Leg

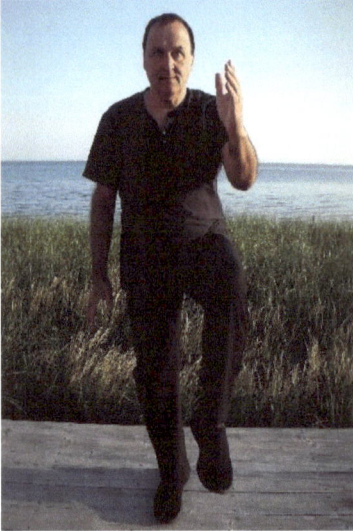

Blending with the previous movement, inhale lifting the left knee, so you are standing on the right leg.

The left elbow is aligned with the left knee fingers pointing to the sky and the palm facing to the side. The right palm extends down the side of the body towards the earth.

On exhalation, lift the left knee a bit more and extend the heel out to the front of the body performing a heel strike. Avoid hyperextending the knee. On inhalation, flex the foot bringing it back to the Standing-on-One-Leg posture. Repeat 3 to 6 times. Practice Relaxed or Reverse Belly Breathing.

7. Extending Front Foot to the Side

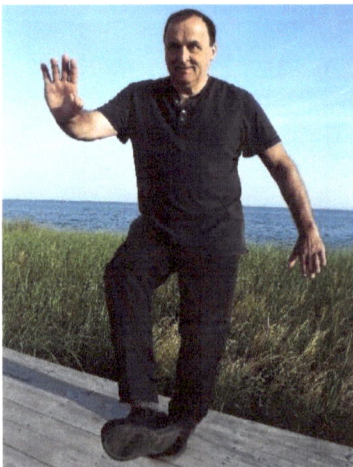

On exhalation, while maintaining the one-legend pose, lower the left leg turning the front foot away from the midline of the body so the sole of the foot faces to the side. The front palm rotates slightly forward.

Hold the posture for 3 to 6 breaths. Practice Relaxed or Reverse Belly Breathing.

This exercise opens the Bladder meridian and helps improve balance.

8. Stepping Back into Coiling Dragon

On exhalation, place the front leg on the ground behind the body into an elongated front stance. The back leg is straight, and the front knee is bent so it tracks above the center of the front foot.

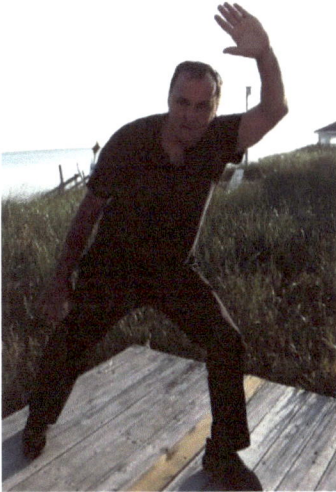

The front palm extends away from the head while the back hand presses in the direction of the rear foot. Both palms are turned outwards, fingers lightly spread apart.

The forward hand is higher than the head. Look to the side. There is a straight line from the back heel to the extended front hand.

You can see the back hand in the peripheral vision. Feel the extension of the body as if you were coiling outwards.

The Coiling Dragon opens the energy pathway of the spinal column and stimulates the central nervous system. Practice Relaxed or Reverse Belly Breathing.

9. Looking Behind to Cure Disease and Injury

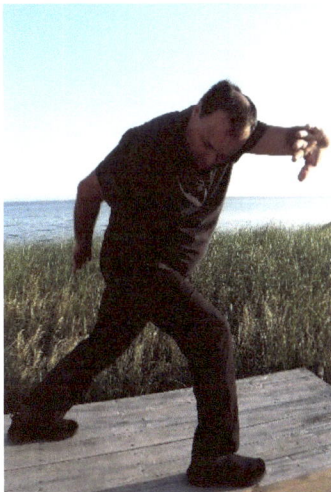

Keeping the same stance, exhale, rotating the trunk towards the front knee, looking back over the shoulder so you can see the back heel.

The front hand extends in the same direction as the spinal rotation about two fist-widths away from the forehead, palm facing out.

The back hand extends behind the lower back, about two fist-widths from the lower back or Ming Men, palm facing out. Hold the posture for a few moments focusing on Relaxed Belly Breathing or Reverse Breathing.

The previous picture shows the exercise with the left leg forward. This picture shows the exercise with the right leg forward. To allow for a smooth transition from Coiling Dragon to the Spinal Twist remain in the left leg forward stance.

10. Modified Extended Side Angle

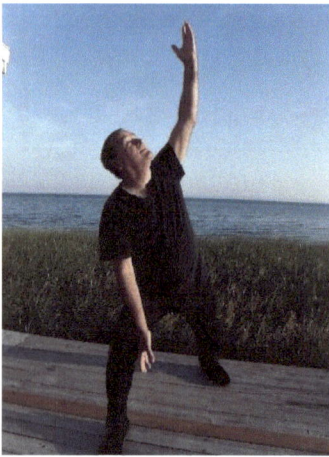

On exhalation, move the back hand down to the inside of the front leg with the palm facing to the side. Raise the other arm up towards the sky. Look up towards the raised hand and breathe into the stretch 3 to 6 times with Relaxed or Reverse Breathing.

Keep the front knee bent so it tracks directly over the center of the front foot and sink the hips down towards the floor. The Modified Extended Angle relieves stiffness in the shoulders and back. It provides a deep groin and hamstring stretch, strengthens the legs and knees, and stretches and strengthens the abdominal muscles.

11. Warrior II Pose

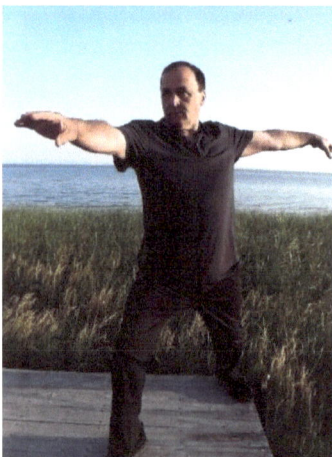

Move from the Modified Extended Side Angle into Warrior II. Simultaneously drop the raised arm and raise the front arm to shoulder height so they are parallel to the earth.

Extend the fingers of both hands far into the distance, dropping the tailbone down towards the earth and opening the Crown Point located on top of the head. Lengthen the stance as you open the hips. Look over the front hand far towards the horizon.

A powerful stretch for the legs, groin, and chest, Warrior II also increases stamina. It helps to relieve backaches and stimulates healthy digestion. This is a deep hip-opening pose that strengthens the thigh and buttock muscles.

Breathe with Natural Belly Breathing or Reverse Breathing for 3 to 6 breaths.

12. Reverse Warrior

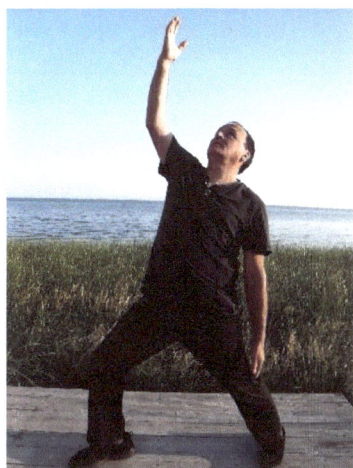

On inhalation, raise the front arm overhead and let the back arm slide down the back leg. Try to keep a light touch on the back leg instead of resting all your weight there. Look up towards the raised hand. The front knee stays deep as the center of the chest opens into a backbend.

Reverse Warrior strengthens and stretches the legs, groins, hips, and the sides of the torso and waist. It improves flexibility in the spine, inner thighs, ankles, and chest. It also builds strength in the thighs, shoulders, and arms.

Breath 6 to 9 times with Relaxed Belly Breathing or Reverse Breathing.

13. One-legged Dragon's Mouth with Humming Hands

To release the body from the previous pose, inhale rotating the trunk to the front with 70% of body weight on the back leg. Move the arms to shoulder height to the front of the body with the palms facing the earth.

Exhale, pulling the body forward with the palms raising the left knee so you are standing on the right leg. Imagine the palms are resting on big energy balloons. Remain in this position for a few moments with Natural Belly Breathing. Feel the Qi beneath the palms.

Inhale with Reverse Breathing bringing Qi to the palms. As you exhale, vibrate the palms with the sound **HHUUMMMMMM**. Repeat 6 to 9 times.

14. Acknowledging the Eight Immortals

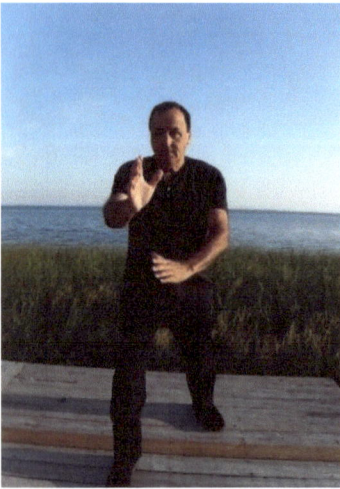

Right Foot Forward

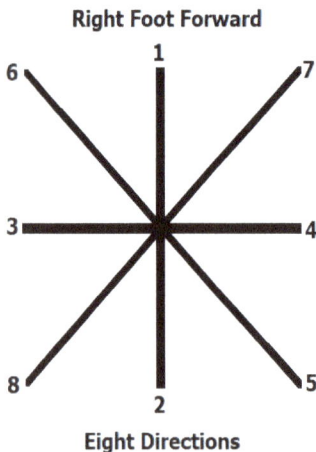

Eight Directions

Inhale with Reverse Belly Breathing. As you exhale, step forward into a front guard posture palms extended forward as if holding a sword into direction number 1. Turn the hips to the front extending Qi out of the palms with eyes opened wide.

Inhale, moving the body weight so it is centered equally between both feet and rotate the body 180 degrees on the balls of the feet, until you face the opposite direction number 2.

At the end of the turn adjust the posture by rotating on the front heel and moving the front foot slightly to the outside to reestablish balance.

Exhale, rotating the hips to the front, shifting the body weight forward, extending Qi out of the palms with eyes opened wide.

Inhale as you turn the hips 90 degrees to position number 3. Exhale stepping forward with the back leg into the front guard posture, rotating the hips to the front.

Shift the body weight forward while extending Qi out the palms with eyes opened wide. Repeat the movement to complete the eight directions as shown in the diagram. The palms are aligned with the center of the body, the front hand is placed at mid-chest height, and the lower hand at navel height. The front hand and front leg move together, and the back hand and back leg move together.

15. Spinning the Sword to Fend Off Danger

Inhale as you step back with the right leg. The opposite arm reaches behind the right shoulder with the palm facing the earth creating a horizontal open-palm sword hand. The other palm extends to the back of the body down towards the earth.

Imagine the left leg is a pole. As you exhale, take three steps around the pole with the right foot rotating the whole body in a 360-degree turn. The sword hand cuts horizontally through the air. The movement ends in a front stance with the right foot at the back and the left foot at the front, both knees slightly bent. The hips drop with the tailbone tilted forward.

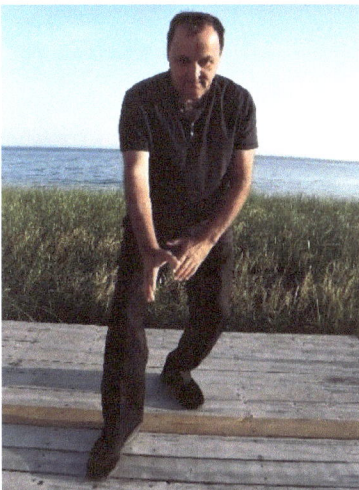

At the completion of the turn both palms rotate up towards the sky, the left leg steps back while the palms cut down the front of the body into a **Tame the Tiger** posture as shown in the picture.

While in this position, imagine you are holding a tiger in front of the body. The inside palm is placed on the lower part of the tigers back while the outside palm is placed just below the neck.

The weight of the body rests mainly on the back foot. The front heel is slightly raised about the width of a pencil. The back leg is full. The front leg is empty. Practice Reverse Belly Breathing.

This movement is an adaptation of an Aikido sword kata. Imagine you are holding a sword in the left hand as the body rotates around its center core fending off evil.

16. Gathering Qi with Reverse Breathing

Inhale with Reverse Belly Breathing letting the body undulate upward with a smooth wavelike motion as the palms reach out the sides of the body towards the sky. The movement starts with the contraction of the abdomen and moves up the body like a wave projecting the arms upward along the sides of the body.

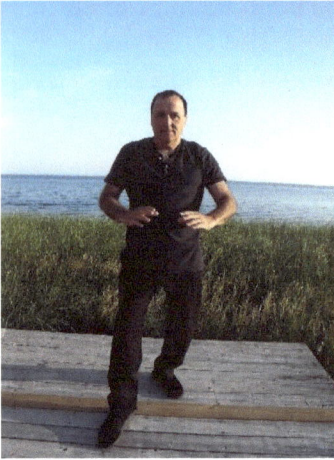

Once the palms are above the head, exhale turning the palms towards the earth and dropping the hands down the center of the body as shown on the picture. Repeat 3 to 9 times before stepping back into the Standing-on-Posts posture arms hanging to the side.

Practice the Eight Diaphragm Breathing Method for about five minutes before repeating the form from the beginning with the focus on the opposite side of the body.

17. Closing Massage with Soong

Refer to the Qi Healers 15-Syle form explained on page 49.

Diagnosing Energy Field Disturbances

An Energy Field Disturbance is the state in which a slowing or blocking of the energy field surrounding a person results in a disharmony of the body, Mind and/or Spirit. In such a case it may be useful to determine if the patient is suffering from a deficient or excess condition. If the patient is suffering from a deficient condition, he or she may need more energy. If a patient is suffering from an excess, balancing or dredging may be required.

In this section we will discuss how to assess the patient's health through:
- Questioning
- Observation of Physical Signs
- Seeing a Disruption in the person's Aura
- Seeing Organs
- Feeling a Disruption through the Palms
- Sensing a Disruption through Whole Body Awareness

Questioning

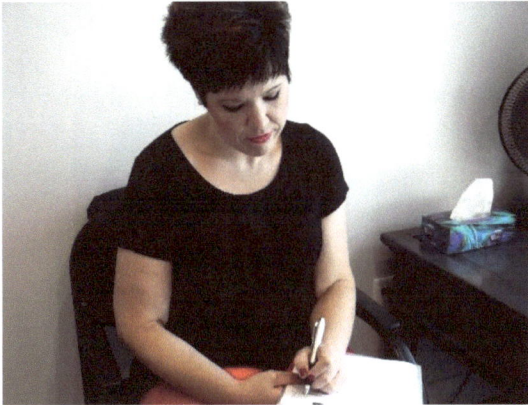

When first meeting a patient, be open minded. Note all first impressions. Identify the major complaints. When and how did they first appear? Identify symptoms experienced mainly within the last six months.

Let the patient speak freely. Look for possible patterns of disharmony. Identify any major injuries, illness or emotional traumas that may have occurred during the patient's life. Has he or she undergone any major operations, suffered from infectious diseases or a long term chronic illness.

Obtain information on the family health history especially of the parents. Is there a family history of a chronic disease? If the parents are deceased, what did they die of?

Questions about emotional traumas experienced by the patient provide some of the most important diagnostic information. Combine the information obtained from asking questions with the other signs and symptoms to help determine the pattern of disharmony. About 80% of illnesses are from internal factors such as emotions and food. The other 20% of illnesses are from accidents and the environment.

Remember that observation takes president over information obtained from the patient.

Observation of Physical Signs

Observation includes looking, hearing, and smelling.

- Looking: Observe the Spirit, demeanor, facial color, body features and how the patient moves.
- Hearing: Listen for the clarity, tone and speed of the voice. Listen to the breathing rhythm, sound, and strength.
- Smelling: Observe any strong, weak or odorless smell on the body or breath. Look for a smell of medications or alcohol. Liver Problems smell like a goat. Heart problems smell like something is burnt. Spleen problems smell fragrant or sweet. Lung Problems smell like fish or a tide pool. Kidney problems smell rotten.

Seeing Auras

A visual person can sometimes see the nuances and shades around the body's energy field generally through the peripheral field of vision. Some highly skilled healers learn to see the colors of the aura, differentiating areas of darkness or light. The colors of the Aura are constantly in motion, reacting to thoughts, feelings, emotional patterns, and environmental influences.

Seeing auras can help identify various diseases and can determine if a person is dying. Normally a bright clear color is an indication of good heath while a turbid, smoky or dark color indicates the presence of disease or disorder.

The colors differ from one section of the body to the other. Since the brain is the center of thoughts and intent, pay special attention to the head area when observing the aura.

Bright white is healthy, smoky white may indicate the onset of disease or artificial stimulation such as drugs, dark and muddy grey indicates potential for health problems, and black represents severe illness or death. Qi Healers often have green energy.

Masters of Qi Gong can open and close their auras. They can close their eyes and still see the different colors of the aura. Most people cannot. To develop these special abilities, train the Mind and have a good Heart. If you practice from the Heart, then the energy grows. You won't get tired. More work equals more kindness, equals more energy.

As you visually scan a patient, look to the sides of the patient's body, observing the silhouette of the outer shell of the patient's Wei Qi or protective energy field. It is important not to stare, but just observe where the field is large, full, thin or broken. Different lighting and backgrounds affect the visual receptivity. The most important characteristic is the clarity of the colors. Observe if the colors are sharp, murky, or concentrated.

Don't treat someone with a black aura radiating from the head. Understand that if person's color is black, you cannot help. There is no need to work. It's the patient's time to leave the world, maybe to go to a better life.

When we are born, we also have a time to die that we can't change. Sometimes a person lives even with a weak body because of **Tao or Virtue,** and sometimes there is a mistake and the person dies ahead of time.

If a patient dies while you are treating them, you will have a problem. Qi Gong can heal many times when a Western Doctor cannot. But normally when a patient dies in the care of a Western Doctor, the legal world does not blame them. It is not the case for energy healers. Qi Healers need to do many, many good things to be accepted. We must be very careful. It is not always good to use your energy for healing.

People who meditate can understand energy. Practice Tao. Be quiet and peaceful. Tao is selfless. Be comfortable with the whole Universe. Even if you do not get along well with the person you are treating, remain comfortable with the healing process. The Heart is the biggest. Be happy. No sadness, no worry, no hurry.

Exercises to Observe the Qi Field

a. Between the Fingers

To practice seeing auras point the index fingers towards each other, palms facing up in front of a dark surface. See the energy stream between the index fingers. Move the fingers side-to-side to enhance it. Then look only at one hand and see energy coming from one finger. Try closing one eye if two do not work. Do not do for too long.

b. Whole Body Aura

Practice seeing the body's energy field around the head and the rest of the body. A partner stands in front of a dark background with eyes closed and expands his or her Qi outward from the body while you use soft eyes to see the aura field. Try closing one eye if two do not work. Do not do for too long

Seeing Organs

In traditional Chinese philosophy, natural phenomena can be classified into the Five Elements: Wood, Fire, Earth, Metal, and Water. These elements are used to describe interactions and relationships between natural phenomena and the body's major organ systems. The Five Element theory describes both a generating cycle and an overcoming or restraining cycle of interactions between the phases.

In the generating cycle:

Liver represents wood which generates fire
Heart represents fire which generates earth
Spleen represents earth which generates metal
Lungs represent metal which generates water
Kidneys represent water which generates wood.

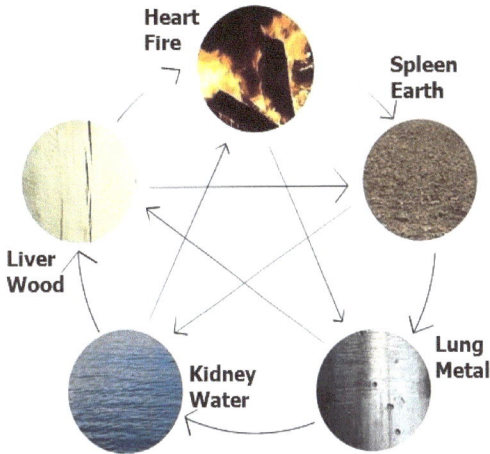

In the overcoming cycle, wood overcomes earth, earth overcomes water, water overcomes fire, fire overcomes metal and metal overcomes wood.

The Five Element Theory can help a Qi Healer diagnose the patient's condition and find appropriate treatments. Through this model we can better understand the Yin and Yang balance in the body organs and apply appropriate corrective treatment to balance Yin and Yang.

For example, if the Heart, which represents Fire, is too Yang meditate on increasing the Kidney Yin, which represents water, to help cool and calm the Heart. If the Heart Fire is too weak meditate on the Liver, which represents wood, to increase its energy and transfer this energy to the Heart. The following are two Qi Gong exercises based on the Five Element Theory.

Seeing the Yin Organs

With practice it is possible to see the color of the internal organs. Imagine a fire ball burning outside of the body. Bring the fire ball in through the mid eyebrow point to the Heart. Meditate on the Heart getting warmer. See the red color of the Heart. Then meditate on each of the other Yin organs, heating the organ to see its color. Follow the organ supporting sequence.

- Heart Fire = Red - Supports Earth or the Spleen
- Spleen Earth = Yellow - Supports Metal or the Lungs
- Lungs Metal = White - Supports Water or the Kidneys
- Kidneys Water = Black or Dark Blue - Supports Wood or the Liver
- Liver Wood = Pearl Green - Supports Fire or the Heart

Harmonize Kidneys and Heart

According to the Five Element Theory the Kidneys represent the Water element and the Heart represents the Fire element. The Kidney Water helps cool or regulate the Heart Fire and the Heart Fire helps heat up the Kidney Water. Each organ system depends on the other to help maintain a state of balance. The following exercise helps regulate the connection between these two organ systems.

Place the left hand above the Heart with the palm facing the chest, about a fist width away from the body. Place the right hand above the Lower Dantian, about a fist width away from the lower abdomen. Breathe naturally for a few minutes, letting the Mind focus on the Heart Fire which is red in color. Then continue breathing for a few minutes letting the Mind focus on the Kidney water which has a dark blue or black color.

Then switch hand positions. For a few minutes focus on cooling the Heart Fire with the Kidney Water and then warming the Kidney Water with the Heart Fire. Switch hands and repeat 3 to 6 times. Switch the hands again and focus on normalizing the Heart Fire and Kidney Water.

Internal Viewing Meditation

The brain can receive and record the vibrations of any object that the senses see, hear, smell, taste or feel. This is also true of thoughts, words and actions. By using light that has a higher vibration than visual light, internal vision sees the energetic flow and structure of the body and the Mind.

After quieting the Mind, imagine the left eye is a bright radiant Sun, while the right eye is a bright and luminous Moon. Join the Sun and Moon light at the Yin Tang or Third Eye Point. As the energies come together they form a bright white ball. This light enters the center of the brain penetrating the pineal gland, which acts as a projector for internal vision.

Next focus your intention on the ball of white light shining down into the body, illuminating the internal organs. Observe and feel the bones, organs and tissue. Allow this information to gather in the Third Eye region. After a while, return to a state of quietness with no Mind allowing these images to settle.

Internal energy viewing helps assess the severity of a disease. The condition of the organs and body tissue can be determined in part by the shade of color they emit. In general, bright clear colors denote a healthy body area while murky, dull, dark colors indicate the presence of a disorder or a disease.

A red or yellow color represents healthy tissue. A dull white color, except for the Lungs which are normally white, may represent the beginning of an energetic dysfunction but is not serious enough to treat. A gray color signifies sickness, while a black color denotes tumors, cancer, or other more serious diseases except for the Kidneys which are normally Black or Dark Blue.

When practicing Internal Viewing do not look for any abnormalities. Let the information appear naturally like a sudden burst of wind, unintended and unexpected. Otherwise you run the risk of imprinting your preconceived ideas on the energy-information being received from the patient.

Palm Scanning

Palm scanning is one of the most common diagnostic methods used by energy healers as the palms are particularly receptive to energy. The person being scanned is lying face up. The healer is on the patient's right side. The patient can also be standing or sitting with feet shoulder-width apart. The patient must be quiet and relaxed.

After adopting a receptive state, the healer focuses on the palm or palms. Do not stare at the palms. The eyes are soft allowing you to see everything in front of you but nothing in particular.

Scan from head to toes with the palms approximately 8 to12 inches away from the body surface. During a scan the palms must be in constant motion. The speed is approximately one foot every two seconds. Scan the person's energy field for openness and symmetry. Move the palms in a smooth and light motion. Focus on the palms which are acting as detectors. They must be relaxed.

- One palm scanning moving the palm from side to side in sections going from head to feet

- Two palms scanning comparing both sides of the body moving from head to feet

- Two palms scanning sweeping out to the sides of the body moving from head to feet

Move the hand to sense a difference. Go on both sides, across, and down the body. Explore the space surrounding the person to find out what is there. Sense the cues to energy imbalance - warmth, coolness, tightness, heaviness, emptiness, tingling or spikes.

Feel the patient's energy looking for differences or anomalies, paying special attention to the organs. The consciousness of the scanner is totally receptive and his or her awareness centered entirely in the hand or hands.

If you scan too fast the Mind does not have enough time to register the sensory input. Too slow and the scanner may feel his or her energy being reflected back. Don't hover too long over one spot as hovering means that you might be giving energy.

Trying to feel the energy tends to block sensory awareness. Allow the sensation of body energies to enter the awareness. Be alert as changes are subtle and may happen quickly even as you are assessing. Identify areas in relation to other parts of the body where the field is different.

You may experience the following:
- Hand moves automatically to an area of the body
- An area of the body pushes the hand out

These are signals that the area needs attention. Pay attention! Remember Auric Diagnosis. If an area is black, don't treat! If it's the Kidney, there is probably no problem as it should be dark.

Normal Organ Indications

Heat	Warm	Red
Kidney	Cool	Black or Dark Blue
Lungs	A bit warm and tingly	White
Stomach	A bit warm	Yellow
Liver	Normal (as other body parts)	Green
Spleen	Normal (as other body parts)	Yellow

Some Abnormal Indications

Temperature Differences - Too warm; Too cold	Usually felt first. Heat = Infections; Cold = Blood Stasis
Pressure	Excess. Dense or Stagnant Energy
Tingling, Needles, Ridges, Spikes	Pain such as Headaches or Migraines
Sharp Needles	Cancer
Heavy, Sticky, or Compacted	Blockages
Hollow, Depletion, Emptiness	Deficiency
Sucking, Grasping, or Pushing	Pulls
Wind	Arthritis or previous surgery
Definite boundaries protecting a vulnerable area.	Armoring

If there is a difference between two sides of the body, correct it. If the whole body seems hot or cold, then it may be you who is disturbed, ill, or out of balance and not the patient. In this situation, use another method, e.g., herbal medicine, acupuncture for example or send the patient to someone else.

Whole Body Diagnosis

Learning to sense the irregularities in a patient's energy field requires compassion, centering and non-attachment. The state of being in which the therapist senses the patient's energy is more important than the actual diagnostic technique. One must be completely in the moment, rooted to the center of the earth and open to the Universe.

The human body emits "bio-fields" of energy that are encoded with information. This information or "message" can be understood by the therapist through energetic resonance indicating the location and severity of the patient's condition.

The energy of the patient and therapist intertwine. Information is exchanged at the energetic level and may express itself in the consciousness of the therapist. This is looking without looking and seeing without seeing.

Whole body diagnosis is done with the patient in the treatment room or at another location. First become quiet, peaceful and relaxed. Extend your energy roots deep into earth and open the Bai Hui or Crown Point. Smile from the Heart. Open the body to the Universe. Be energetically rooted and transparent.

Create an energetic resonance with the patient. Take a snap shot looking at the overall picture with your inner vision. Let the image settle in your consciousness.

It is important to get a clear picture of the person before proceeding to treatment. Images or impressions may suddenly appear instantaneously without warning. Note any Qi deviations.

Once the condition of the patient becomes apparent, the therapist sends healing messages to the person encoded in the Qi. Using the Mind, the therapist clears the dense Qi, smooths the pain ridges, and infuses the patient with vibrant Qi.

The therapist must have secure emotional boundaries. Otherwise he or she may project their own feelings onto the patient or may inadvertently absorb the patient's pathogenic energy.

Recognize with whom you are dealing. What is appropriate for one person may not be for another.

- **Very Sensitive** – Do not touch. Sit connected with the Universe and talk. Words can heal.
- **Cannot Find Any Problems** – General dredging and sending of energy.
- **Patient wants more energy** – Give no more as they already have what they need.
- **If you are feeling challenged,** ask your teacher or school for help.

Secrets of External Qi Healing

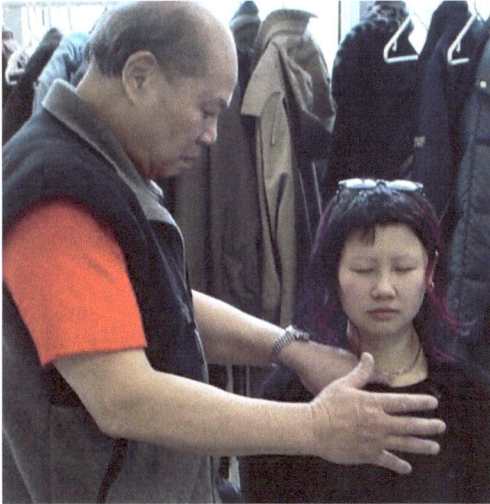

All diseases have a Yin and a Yang aspect. Yang is the outside energy, Yin is the inside manifestation. Even cancer has a Yin and Yang aspect. Allopathic medicine gives a substance to ingest, which kills the Yin or takes it out. Then one doesn't feel the Yang. The Qi Healer does the opposite. We take away the Yang or outside energy, then the Yin rebalances as Yin cannot exist without Yang.

Qi healing is not invasive. We are affecting the external energy field. The internal energy depends upon the external field, so as we correct the external, the internal changes and corrects itself. This is not magic. We correct an area and make it comfortable by correcting Qi circulation, level, evenness and temperature.

Qi healing is not harmful. A surgeon must not fumble. A Qi Healer can fumble. Why? Because a scalpel has much less intelligence than Qi. Qi is an informational substance that knows where to go and what to do to rebalance the body's energy.

Qi Healers are not alone when they do treatments as they benefit from an open channel to their teachers. In turn, the teacher has an open channel to his masters (Confusion, Taoist, Buddhist, Medical) so our energy comes from that lineage. Call on you teacher and the Eight Immortals for assistance in healing.

The Eight Immortals have long been part of Chinese history. They represent a group of eight celestial beings that are believed to know the secrets of nature. They represent separately male, female, the old, the young, the rich, the noble, the poor, and the humble Chinese. Each of the individual immortal's power can be transferred to a tool of power that can give life or destroy evil.

In Qi healing, you can you give too much Qi. You can fix the body with Qi and obtain balance. But then if you continue the body will become unbalanced. If the patient already feels good, then there is no need to continue. Unbalanced is uncomfortable. If you give balanced energy there is no problem.

Keep the Mind on **"give and get out."** Both directions are important. If a person is weak, they may feel dizzy because of the "out." So we must maintain a balance. After treating, always give energy to the patient. Often results from treatment occur about 24 hours after the Qi healing is done, but sometimes immediately.

During treatment, take care not to even think about "bad" energy, as it will come to you. Just think "I want to help this person and I can do it!" You are a healer, and you can help your patient!

Also, when you get rid of toxic energy say "Deep under the ground!" not "Next door!" for the energy taken out must be disposed of properly. Don't merely flick it away. Think it down, to the center of the earth! Or else you will be able to feel the cold spots on the floor. Sometimes it slips away like mercury and is difficult to get rid of and flies around the room like a bird. If you do make a mistake, you must get the toxic energy out using the Mind.

Energy comes from the Mind to build Qi and heal others. When doing Qi Healing these are important points to remember:

- Remain centered, quiet, peaceful, and relaxed
- The patient must be open to receive Qi Healing
- Create the right atmosphere
- Understand the problem
- Send the right Qi
- Qi follows the Mind
- Mind creates reality and effect
- When Qi is focused it gathers Essence, substance will be formed, physical change will occur
- Heal Heart to Heart

- Qi is the most powerful tool to heal others
- With the correct Mind all else will fall into place
- Never underestimate the importance of good character

Pain and disease come mainly from negative emotions. Remember that Qi works on emotions.

When is Qi Gong most effective?

- Prevention: While we are still well, to keep us well. For ourselves and others.

- Early Stages of Disease: When the first symptoms appear - sub-clinical, long before we would ordinarily go to the doctor.

- Middle Stages of Illness: Often working in conjunction with other therapies and physicians.

- Late Stages of Illness: To ease pain and fear when death is imminent.

Qi Gong can help with many conditions such as healing bones more quickly - sometimes very quickly - old painful injuries; panic attacks; anxiety; stress and all dysfunctions it causes; chronic pain; fatigue; organ (Dysfunction / Exhaustion / Infection); endocrine imbalances; bleeding; first aid to injuries (even grave injuries); Heart and Blood pressure disorders, and many more.

The Qi finds all the roots and seeds of the disorder and neutralizes them. The Qi has intelligence and will go where it must for the healing.

The highest Qi Gong has no shape and no direction. Form does not matter, *it already worked!* An experienced practitioner can even slouch and still be effective in doing Qi Gong healing.

External Qi Healing Methods

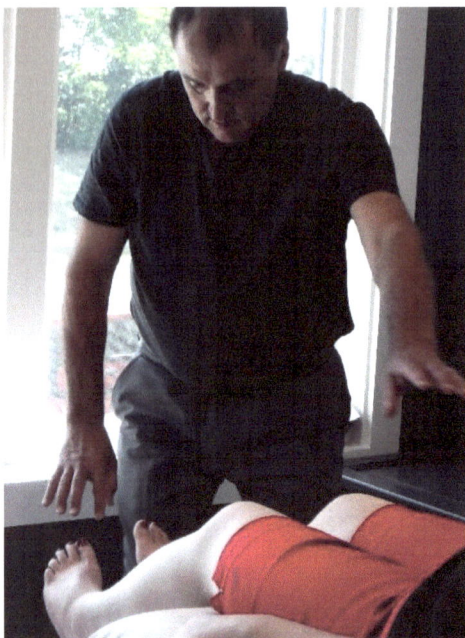

Qi Healing treatments may last anywhere from five minutes to 45 minutes. The length of treatment depends on factors such as the condition being treated, the patient's receptivity to treatment, and the healing modalities available to the therapist.

Independently of the problem being treated, we first correct our own Mind. Relax, then we can move energy. The therapist creates an environment of confidence that allows the patient to relax. Enter the patient's energy field with confidence and softness, as any rough or quick movement may create more pain and discomfort.

The therapist must understand his/her patients and know what to talk about to make them feel happy. When we are happy we build more energy. Help the patient focus on something nice outside of the body. If patient is Yin, talk Yang. If Yang, talk Yin. For example, a headache is Yang so talk about a beautiful lake.

For patients who cannot relax, who have a quick beating Heart, not enough Blood in the Heart, we can help them slow down with one of the following exercises:

Counting Breath: On inhalation the patient counts silently to seven. On exhalation the patient counts to 10. There is no need to remember the count. This strengthens the Dantian energy situated in the lower abdomen and strengthens the Kidneys and Bladder.

Abdominal Breathing: Inhale through the nose, expanding the abdomen. Exhale letting the abdomen return to its original position. Inhale 70% of respiratory capacity and exhale 100%.

Listen to the empty space after exhalation and let the inbreath rise on its own.

Dantian Breathing:

- Breathe into the Upper Dantian 6 to 9 times via the Mid-Eyebrow Point
- Breathe into the Middle Dantian 6 to 9 times via the Mid-Chest Point
- Breathe into the Lower Dantian 6 to 9 times via the Gate of Qi point located about two to three finger widths below the navel

During the first part of the exercise, the therapist can help the patient become aware of the location of the points by gently placing his or her fingers on each energy center.

Different Types of Energetic Intervention

The major objectives of treatment are to break up and clear out stagnant Qi, smooth ruffled Qi to help it flow more smoothly, and build strong Qi. This is achieved through several methods such as Opening the Energy Gates, Fa Qi with Magic Palm, Sword Fingers, Immortal Single Grasp Method, Spiraling Energy Method, Chakra Clearing, Whole Body Dredging, Smoothing the Qi Method, Buda Palms and Mind Clearing.

All methods rely on the Mind to direct the Qi and provide it with purpose. Some techniques include movement of the hands at a distance. Others use light touch and little or no physical movement.

Spiraling Energy Method

The Spiraling Energy Method can be used to open and close the patient's energy field at the beginning and end of a treatment. It connects all major chakras and can also be used to open energy centers or build Qi at a specific location.

To open the energy field at the beginning of a treatment, with the patient supine on the treatment table, place the left palm about 10 to 12 inches above the chest center. Pause for a moment focusing on opening the Heart energy. Moving in a counter clockwise direction, spiral the palm over the upper chest to the Solar Plexus, throat, Yellow Court (Just below the sternum), Yin Tang, Qi Hai, Bai Hui, root chakra, and transpersonal point located just above the crown of the head. You may pause for a moment at each point.

It is important to focus the Mind on opening the patient's energy field. Normally, to open the energy field, spiral in a counter clockwise direction. At the end of treatment reverse the procedure and direction of the spiral to close the energy field. Focus the mind on closing the energy field.

The counter-clockwise Spiraling Energy Method can also be used to open chakras or acupoints while clockwise spiraling is used to energise these same points.

Opening the Energy Gates

The Opening of the Energy Gates Sequence is a full body intervention that helps balance the patient's major energy centers thus making the person more receptive to treatment. It also harmonizes the body's energy field, enhances the flow of Qi, and produces a sense of deep relaxation and awareness.

The healer is sitting or standing at the side of the patient. The technique is normally applied with a combination of light touch and hands held at a distance from the patient depending on which area of the patient is being treated. The hands move from one energy center to the other in the following order:

- Yong Quan Kid 1 - Soles of Feet and Ankles
- Ankle and Knees
- Knee and Hips
- Hips or Hui Yin (Pelvic Floor)
- Root Chakra and Qi Hai (Below Navel)
- Qi Hai and Solar Plexus
- Solar Plexus and Dan Zhong (Mid Chest)
- Dan Zhong and Throat
- Throat and Yin Tang (Mid Eyebrow Point)
- Yin Tang and Bai Hui (Crown Point)
- Bai Hui or Crown Point
- Transpersonal Point (About a foot above the head)

Begin by gently holding both feet with the hands for about a minute to help bring the energy down to the feet. Use both hands, or alternating hands as you move up the body. Hold or hover above each point until you feel a shift in the energy or for 1 to 3 minutes. Use the Mind to spin each point in a clockwise or counter-clockwise direction until the area under your palms feels balanced.

Chakra Clearing

Chakra clearing opens and normalizes Chakra energy and helps treat severe pain. Start the treatment in the energy field located above the Crown Chakra and work your way gradually down to the feet. The patient can be lying on their back or sitting in a chair.

Place the palms in the energy field above the crown of the head, palms facing away from each other. Gently and slowly spread both hands outward as far as   comfortably. Repeat this movement three times.

Spread the palms outward over each Chakra in a similar fashion in the following order: Transpersonal Point, Crown Point, Mid Eyebrow, Throat, Heart, Solar Plexus, Qi Hai, Hui Yin and Root Chakra. Notice how each Chakra feels.

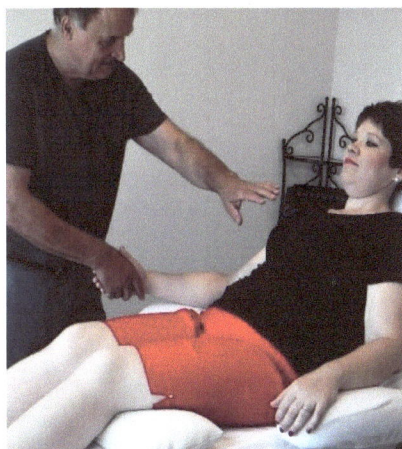

Continue by spreading the energy centers around the knees and ankles. End by dredging the lower legs and sending the energy deep into the earth.

During the treatment, if the patient releases strong emotions help the person stay calm by holding their hand in a thumb lock position for about a minute hovering the other palm over the Heart area.

Whole Body Clearing

This method clears the whole body of congested energy balancing the energy field.

The patient lies on a table on the back. The therapist begins by placing their hands about 12 inches above the patient's head, palms facing towards the head, fingers pointing down like rakes.

Use a long continuous raking motion starting above the head and moving down the center of the body to the feet. The movement is continuous and smooth coming off the body beyond the toes. As you rake imagine you are clearing the energy body of dense Qi.

Move slowly from head to feet repeating three to five times. Then switch sides for comfort. Dredge the center as well as both sides of the body. The fingers are reaching deep into the body.

The palms face the healer coming back. The treatment can last from 5 to 10 minutes or until the energy feels smooth and even. Release any stagnant Qi deep into the centre of the earth.

This technique is good for addictions, fibromyalgia, chronic systemic disease, post chemo and radiation, post surgery, MS and Parkinson.

Fa Qi with Magic Palm, Laser Fingers and Sword Hand

Often during a Qi Gong workshop, the instructor sends out Qi to all the participants using Magic Palm. The palms can be used both to feel and to extend Qi. The objective when extending Qi can be to break up stagnation, release toxic Qi from the body, move the Qi between two points, smooth ruffled Qi, or build strong Qi in the Lower Dantian.

The Mind is used to provide direction and intent to the Qi while pushing and pulling the Qi with the palms. By adding a spiraling motion, the palms can be used to strengthen the Qi in a weakened area of the body or to release stagnant Qi.

Spiral the hand in a clockwise direction to augment the intensity of the Qi and in a counter clockwise direction to open the area, reduce the Qi, break up congested areas and reduce pain. A back and forth movement helps to smooth ruffled Qi improving its flow.

Three hand positions can be used depending on what type of Qi is required to help the patient. The three hand positions are the Magic Palms with focus on the palm center, laser fingers with the focus on the tips of the fingers, and Sword Hand. (Thumb pressed on the outside of the nails of the 4th and 5th fingers, and the index and ring fingers pointing forward).

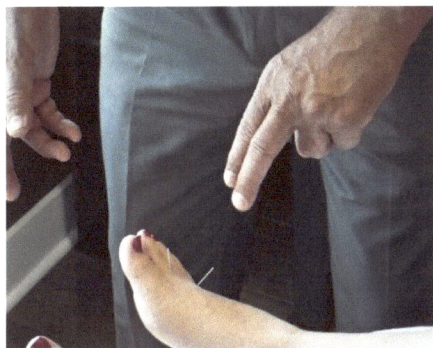

The open palm covers a greater area with a more general focus. The laser fingers and Sword Hand provide a more focused energy beam used to penetrate deeper into the body on smaller areas to break up tumors or congestion along the body's meridians or energy pathways. The Sword Hand, as seen in the picture, can be used to activate Qi in acupuncture needles.

When treating a patient with Magic Palm, Laser Fingers or Sword Hand imagine a laser beam extending out from the palm or fingers. A raking or back-and-forth motion can be used with Laser Fingers or Sword Hands to cut up and release stagnant Qi.

Smoothing the Qi Field

This technique is used for smoothing or balancing the Qi in the meridians, unruffling pain ridges and sealing wounds. This technique releases dense Qi so the energy flows more smoothly. Good for migraines, digestive issues and tension headaches.

To unruffle pain ridges repeatedly sweep the hands from above to below the site. Do this for three to five minutes noting any change in the energy field.

A wound or energy leak may feel like a column of cool air pushing against the hand. To seal a wound gather energy from the affected area moving the palms back and forth over the wound or energy leak. Then to seal the leak hold the palm over the area for about a minute.

Rescan for other leaks until the treated area feels smooth like the rest of the body.

This technique can also be used to move the Qi in a meridian or between two points on the body. Place the palms at opposite ends of a congested area and use the Mind to move the Qi between these points much like the movement of a bubble in a carpenter's level. You can also visualise an open connection between the two points.

The Qi Healer can also move the palms back and forth, or up and down between two points over a congested area until it feels open and light.

Immortal Single Grasp Method

This technique is used to take out the pathogenic energy from the body. It clears out specific areas of stagnation.

Scan the body with the palms. When you find a congested area, close the fingers around the toxic Qi. Use a claw-like hand or Iron Tong to pluck out the pathogenic or overactive energy with profound understanding.

Move the hand at least two feet away from the body. Open the hand. Send pathogenic Qi into the center of the earth. Pull out toxic Qi three times sending it deep into the earth. Reach in, pull out, cast down deep into the earth with exhalation.

Using palm scanning, redo the diagnosis. As the condition improves, the feeling becomes lighter.

Do not use this technique if the pregnant women does not feel comfortable with it.

Buda Palm

This is a whole-body method that is useful when there are several problems occurring in different areas of the body. Buda Palm is good for chronic conditions. It balances the whole body!

When working in a more defined area, use the Immortal Single Grasp Method to take out the stagnant Qi.

The patient is lying on their back. Meditate with the teacher and the Universe for a few moments. Diagnose the body using the palms, Whole-Body Sensing, or auric sight.

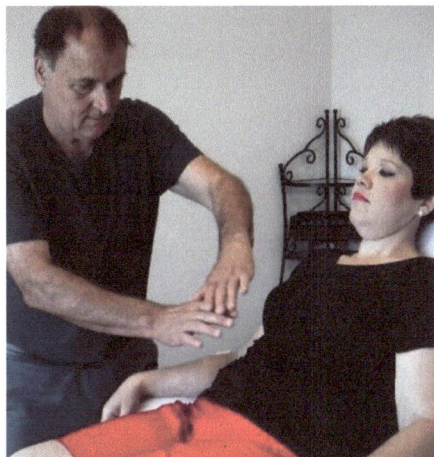

To cleanse the patient's body of toxic Qi, inhale with Natural Belly Breathing while running the back of hands up the side of the patient's body. The palms are facing away from the patient. Move the hands from below the feet to above the head.

Above the Bai Hui turn the palms down. Exhale, emitting Qi while moving the hands from the Bai Hui down over center of body to below the feet. With the palms as least two feet away from the patient, mentally bury the pathogenic Qi deep into the center of the earth. Repeat for 3 to 6 times.

Reread or diagnose the patient. If the energy is not balanced repeat the above method. If the energy is normal, strengthen and store the Qi in the patient's Lower Dantian.

To strengthen Qi in the Lower Dantian, inhale while running the backs of hands up the center of the patient's body to the Upper Dantian. Exhale, turning the palms over and moving them down to face the Lower Dantian. The palms face the Lower Dantian in a diamond shape. Rotate the palms 100 times in a clockwise direction to reinforce the Jing Qi. This helps restore vitality.

Pause the movement and breathe in Universal energy via the Crown Point, soles of the feet and Hui Yin into the Lower Dantian. Exhale and extend the Qi via the palms into the patient. Repeat 10 to 12 times. Then gently remove the hands from the energy field and step away from patient.

One never gets tired using this method, because it is Qi Gong practice for the therapist as well as healing for the patient.

Breathe naturally. Always say, think and believe that you want to help this person and always know that it works. When taking out toxic Qi or mingling with the patient's Qi, don't fear, doubt or pause for a second as toxic energy will come into you.

Use your Mind with Universal energy and the teacher's energy. You may also want to call on the energy of the Eight Immortals if you need an extra energy boost with a specific patient.

Mind Clearing

This technique relaxes the patient, focusing and clearing the Mind of excessive thoughts. During this process, you can also use the Mind to do distant healing on the patient.

For best results, the patient lays on a treatment table on the back so the head area is accessible. The Qi Healer sits at the head of the table and places their fingers gently on the shoulders of the patient. Relax and hold the position for about three minutes.

Then move the fingers slowly to the mid neck area, the occipital area, then to the area on the scull just above the ears. Hold each area for about three minutes. With the finger pads resting on the area just above the ears, let the thumb pads drop and rest on the crown of the head for about 3 minutes.

Place the palm of one hand under the occipital ridge. Then gently place the finger pads of the free hand just above the eyebrows and pull the finger pads gently towards the patient's hair line. Repeat 3 to 6 times.

Place the finger pads on the temples and practice Whole Body Sensing to discover any congested areas of the body that need treatment.

If required use the Mind to cleanse, regulate or strengthen the Qi field of the patient. Use the breath to smooth out energetic ridges, break up congestion, cool warm areas or warm cool areas. Then gently release the physical contact and energetic bond.

Distant Healing

Distant healing allows you to heal at a distance with the patient in the same room or at another location. During treatment, the healer shifts into a healing meditation state that facilitates the energy transfer between the practitioner and the recipient as well as the repatterning of the patient's energy field through the process of resonance.

Bring the Mind into focus. If you need help think of your teacher and more energy will come. The Mind is used to give intent and direction to the Qi. Moving of the hands can provide some help in focusing the intent.

First still the body, and quiet the Mind. If you are in the same room as the patient, on inhalation, let pure Universal energy enter your Crown Point, moving down the center core of the body to the Lower Dantian.

On exhalation, drop the energy down to the feet. Then let it bounce back up expanding outward encompassing the healer's and the patient's energy fields. The energy remains anchored and the body transparent.

Sense the patient's energy and any blockages that may be present in the person's energy field. Clean out pathogenic Qi and balance the energy flow. Remain emotionally neutral throughout the whole process.

If working at a distance, picture the patient in your Mind. Sense the patient's energy and any blockages. Clean out pathogenic Qi and balance the energy flow. Visualize the patient getting better.

Remain energetically transparent and emotionally neutral throughout the whole process. When the treatment is complete, disconnect from the patient's energy field, and rest the Mind in the Lower Dantian for a few moments.

The priority in distance healing is for the Qi Healer to establish a connection between the three Dantians through the absorption of Universal Qi into the Tai Chi Pole. Once this connection is established, the Qi Healer initiates the whole-body connection with the patient. Once the therapist feels the connection the treatment may begin.

During treatment, the therapist may play a more passive role letting the energy go where it needs to go to balance the person's Qi.

Or the therapist may be more active in directing the Qi, visualizing the patient's pathogenic energy dispersing and melting away deep into the ground. The therapist may visualize dark areas becoming brighter, hot areas becoming cooler or cold areas becoming warmer.

During the treatment the body manifests what the Mind believes and the Heart feels. After normalizing and energizing these areas, the therapist withdraws the projected Shen or Spirit back into the body disconnecting from the patient's energy field.

Difficult Cases

A patient may need only one treatment to fix a problem. But ask the patients to come three to five times to provide a follow-up to treatment and ensure it has worked to the patient's satisfaction. Book treatments once or twice a week for 3 to 5 weeks.

Teach patients the importance of a healthy diet and lifestyle, a tranquil Mind, and positive emotions. Emotional problems may stem from the brain. Therefore, treat the brain like you would the Liver or other organ systems.

Get feedback from the patients during treatment. You may be moving too slow or too fast for them to feel better. Keep a fairly slow and even pace in the movements because energy needs to move, and "get out". The patient may not feel the energy shift if the movements are too fast. If the person being treated feels nothing, consider giving them another type of treatment.

When taking out toxic Qi and it burns, the pathogenic energy is too strong for you. If you feel confident, rub your hands together to make more energy. There is no need to work too hard. With more energy, it is easier to get into the other person's energy field as energy flows from the strong to the weak, or like water from the high point to the low point.

This is the reason why a Qi Healer needs to develop and maintain strong Qi. The healer must also recognise their strengths and weaknesses. If the therapist suffers from a chronic Lung disorder, he or she may succumb more readily to the pathogenic Qi of patients suffering from a Lung problem.

When a patient comes to you for treatment and you are not feeling well, or your energy is low, and referring the patient to another Qi Healer is not an option, send energy to the Kidney points. The Kidneys can never have enough energy. Energizing the Kidneys makes all body organs feel good.

Some Difficult-to-Treat Conditions:

- Spiritual based
- Medicated people
- Past life issues
- Recurring environmental
- Surgery

There are three additional methods for patients who feel Qi.

1. Meditate and call on your teacher and the Eight Immortals to help in the healing process. Use this method only if you don't have enough energy to cure the person.

- Respect the teacher
- Meditate on the face, voice or energy of the teacher
- Remain quiet and peaceful. Open the Qi door and grow your energy. Then you can do it.

Think of the teacher, all your teachers, especially their energy. Invoke their help. Do this until your palms feel warm and full indicating that the body has more energy. Then work. You are now using the energy you gathered and that of the teacher's.

It's not right to ask the teacher for help every time -- this doesn't respect the teacher. If you always ask, later, you won't be able to do the work yourself. Invoke the teacher's help only when you really need it.

2. If don't know how to fix a problem, just do it. Just ask what the problem is and say "I can do it!" Believe! Qi has intelligence and will go where it is needed.

3. The problem is already fixed. If the patient is very sensitive, you just need a good Mind. You don't need movement. Just use Mind work and the problem will be fixed from just the good words. The patient is healed because you say it is so as words heal for sensitive patients.

Dealing with Toxic Energy

Both of my Qi Gong instructors shared a common vision on how to deal with Toxic Qi. Qi can build or destroy. Toxic Qi can jump into the healer while doing a Qi Healing treatment. It may hide in the Qi Healer's body only manifesting itself after several years as the healer's immune system weakens.

To protect yourself against toxic Qi, above all, remember the importance of virtue. Be kind. You must have a good Mind and a good Heart. Fear, anger, guilt or desire will deplete your energy. Extreme emotions can throw us off track. The way we think has a strong impact on our emotions.

We lose Qi if we are angry, jealous, or have a lack of confidence in ourselves or others. If we worry or are afraid we lose Qi. There are many reasons to be angry. Do not get so angry so it comes from the Heart. Extreme emotions – too angry, too happy, too sad – weaken Qi.

You need to be happy for energy to come. A happy Mind is open. Sad energy goes out and down. Fear energy contracts. Tension and worry energy tightens. Anxiety energy raises up and agitates. No need to worry, to hurry or to get angry. Be happy, relaxed and peaceful. This will balance the energy in whole body. With a correct Mind, Heart and Spirit, the body will be healthier.

Smile with everything. Be happy with everything. Enjoy life and get energy. The body's energy needs to circulate. If there is too much tension the energy doors will close.

Strong Qi is required to disperse pathogenic energy. You can never have too much Qi, thus the importance of practicing energy cultivation techniques.

Pathogenic or toxic Qi can come from external sources. When the immune system is low, external injuries or negative influences can cause blockages. We do not know when pathogenic Qi will enter the body.

We cannot overstate the importance of practicing Qi Gong to strengthen resistance to disease and allow Qi to pass through the blockages. There is less chance of being sick, less chance of external pathogenic Qi entering the body when the Qi is strong.

Tension starts when we are born when we cry for food and love. As we get older we think too much. We get caught up in jealousy and competition. If your Mind is not happy, it creates tension. Many energy doors close.

We need lots of love, a Heart that can receive everything. We must work on our character and emotions to have better Qi. We must spend time with what makes us happy.

A little smile on the face works magic. Let the eyebrows drop and mouth relax. The Yin Tang or mid-eyebrow point opens connecting the Heart and Brain. Smile from the Heart. This helps avoid a buildup of toxic Qi.

To protect yourself:

- Have a good and compassionate Heart
- Develop strong Qi by practicing Qi Gong
- Think of yourself as a healer. Do not be scared or pathogenic Qi will affect you.

We must understand that we are complete. Be always happy and your energy will always be open. Someone is mad at you and you are still happy. Believe in yourself and you will do good for society.

Treatment Tips

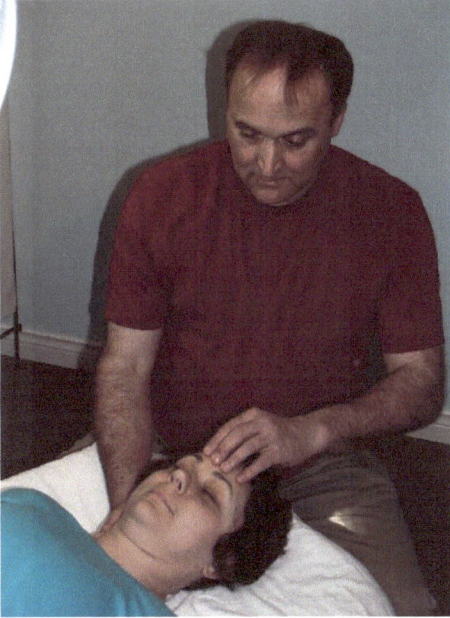

Qi Healing techniques are taught individually but when doing Qi Healing, follow your intuition and choose the technique or combination of techniques that best correspond to the ever-changing energy patterns of the patient.

During treatment, the healer shifts into a healing meditation state that:
- Increases the sensitivity of the healer to the patient's energy
- Facilitates the energy transfer between the practitioner and the recipient
- Facilitates the repatterning of the patient's energy field through the process of resonance.

Energetic Assessment

It is important to continually reassess the patient's energy to determine the effects of treatment and to adapt to the changing state of the patient's energy field. Look for any abnormalities in the energy field such as pulls, pushes, wind, cold, hot, ruffles, voids, vibration, prickling sensation, or pins and needles. Most importantly listen to your inner wisdom and follow your intuition.

Treatment

Focus the intent on the re-patterning of areas of imbalance and blocked Qi. The intensity of the energy flow can be influenced by imagery and breath which can help move the Qi, as well as by using various hand positions and movement. The normal sequence is to clear energy blockages, smoothe the flow of Qi, and strengthen the patient's Dantian energy.

Grounding of Patient

After treatment, disconnect from the patient's energy field and let the person rest for a few minutes to help integrate the effects of the treatment. Then bring the patient back by touching the feet. Separate your field from theirs. Check their eyes to make sure they are awake. Offer them water. Wash your hands and forearms.

Evaluation and Feedback

Ask the patient to provide feedback to help evaluate the effectiveness of treatment and validate your impression of the state of the person's energy field.

Home Care

Offer referrals if appropriate, home care, and additional treatments. Document the session for future reference.

There are many home care exercises that can be prescribed to the patient. They all start with some form of meditation to help the person become quiet, peaceful and relaxed. As most problems are emotionally based, being quiet, peaceful and relaxed brings more energy to help resolve these issues.

We can teach patients:

- Posture: How to sit, stand, walk and lay down.
- Healthy lifestyle to help correct their condition.
- Proper breathing to help the patient relax and calm the Mind
- The importance of movement for health and wellness as embodied in some forms of Yoga, Tai Chi or Qi Gong.

Treatment Sequence

The healer's ability to center is the basic tool for all energetic interventions. Centering is the focused intent that is required to connect with Universal energy. In addition, the healers physical body needs to be relaxed, the emotions calm, the Mind clear, and the Spirit quiet and still.

1. Prepare the Client and the Environment

- Provide privacy and a relaxing atmosphere
- Establish a trusting relationship

2. Observation

- Observe the way the person walks, their posture, their complexion, their breath, the tone of their voice, and the quality of their Spirit (Eyes).

3. Questioning / Update

- Identify client's main reason for coming
- Obtain clients consent to treatment
- Update information as needed from previous sessions if required.

4. Prepare Client

- Explain energy healing
- Ask permission to touch if part of treatment
- Give permission to the client to stop treatment at any time
- The patient may be treated sitting, standing or lying down comfortably on their back.
- The patient must be quiet, peaceful and relaxed. Instruct he/her how to breathe from the abdomen. You may recommend the Three Dantian Breathing exercise.

5. Grounding and Centering of Therapist

- Center the body and the Mind by rooting the body to the earth. Open the body to the Universe. Smile from the Heart.

6. Open the Energy Field

- Connect to the patient's energy field with heartfelt compassion.
- You may decide to do a preliminary dredging to clear the body and relax the patient
- Maintain a compassionate and caring attitude

7. Energetic Assessment

- Sense the energy in the palms
- Scan from head to feet

- Use constant motion while moving through the energy field
- Move at a speed of one foot per two seconds
- Keep the palms eight to 12 inches away from the body surface
- Look for disharmonies in the energy field

Other assessment methods may be used independently or jointly with palm scanning such as Seeing the Aura, Seeing the Organs or Whole-Body Sensing.

8. Transfer of Symptoms

- Recognize how you feel that day to be able to identify issues that do not belong to you
- Recognize when it is not your issue but the patients
- If you encounter problems step back and reconnect with the Universe
- Be professional. Do not take on other people's problems. They're not yours.

9. Practical Tips:

- Remove jewelry
- Wear loose, comfortable clothing
- Practice in a clean, well-ventilated environment
- Healer keeps eyes open or half closed. The patient may keep their eyes closed
- Do not administer Qi Healing with pregnant or ill patients: Cold, flu, severe infection.
- The recipient must ask or at least be open to energy healing unless incapacitated by a stroke, a coma or another condition
- Know your limitations. Make referrals to licensed healthcare practitioners whenever necessary.

Summary of Important Points

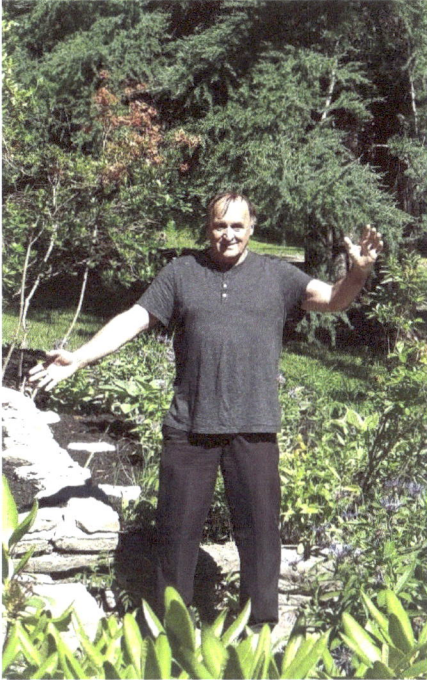

The healer must be balanced. If the healer is not good in Mind and deeds, there will be no healing energy. Relax the body. The Mind must be peaceful. Focus and use breath.

After giving Qi, and during the treatment, keep warm as you are very open. After giving healing energy, you will feel like you have done Qi Gong. You have! Feel the energy. Smile to the energy. Give the energy to someone else. Feel more energy.

Never think about the patient's problem or toxic energy. Just concentrate on giving energy correctly. Your Mind must discipline the energy - throw away toxic energy briefly and quickly. This keeps toxic energy from entering the healer. If for some reason you did not throw toxic energy away firmly, it can be like a bird in the room. Catch it and throw it away again.

Be aware of the direction of energy between you and the patient. Your energy should be flowing to the patient as your energy is STRONGER than the patient's energy.

To keep the patient comfortable and to protect yourself from toxic Qi, always guide the pathogenic energy down deep into the earth. Keep testing and checking adjusting your treatment accordingly. Always give energy after a test.

If you have a difficult condition to treat, it is okay to give the patient a massage first to open and loosen the body. Then use energy to clear and energize.

The safest technique is extraction. If you have doubts about what to do, just test and take out stagnant Qi via the Immortal Single Grasp Method. If a person is weak, do not take out too much energy through the feet as it may weaken the person further.

Conditions that require further training:

Cancer, breaking up stones, deafness, and muscle spasticity are some of the most difficult conditions to treat.

1. Do not treat mental illness
2. Do not treat a patient with schizophrenia
3. Do not touch the patient sexually or act seductively

For pregnant women or for women who are having a period use Magic Palms. Do not do full body dredging as this strongly guides the energy down and out. If the problem is localized in the uterus do not treat! Sometimes you may use Mind Clearing. Practice virtue or there'll be no energy.

For Children, it is best to use Qi. They are open to it. If child is 1-2 months old, there is no need for treatment.

Do not practice Qi Gong or do energy healing in a windy, wet, cold, or hot environment.

In Qi Gong train the Spirit and the Body with:

- No thoughts
- Mind in the Lower Dantian
- Focus the Mind on the point or area of blockage

If you have a good Heart you will have energy to help people. Qi Healers can fix problems that come from unbalanced emotions because they can release blocked energy caused by emotional trauma. By removing the energy blockages emotions will flow again and the emotional-related pain will disappear.

Qi Healers must practice Qi Gong regularly to relax more and make their energy denser. Practice too little and the water won't boil (need at least 20 minutes a day). Practice too much and the water or Qi will boil away.

If you give something, it must be from the Heart. If you feel afterwards that you gave too much, you will lose energy. In the beginning, we open the Mind, see the blockages, and circulate energy. At later levels of practice, there will be no need to see. You will just know.

Practice no hurry, no worry. Smile from the Heart. Be happy like the Dragon Dancing in the Universe.

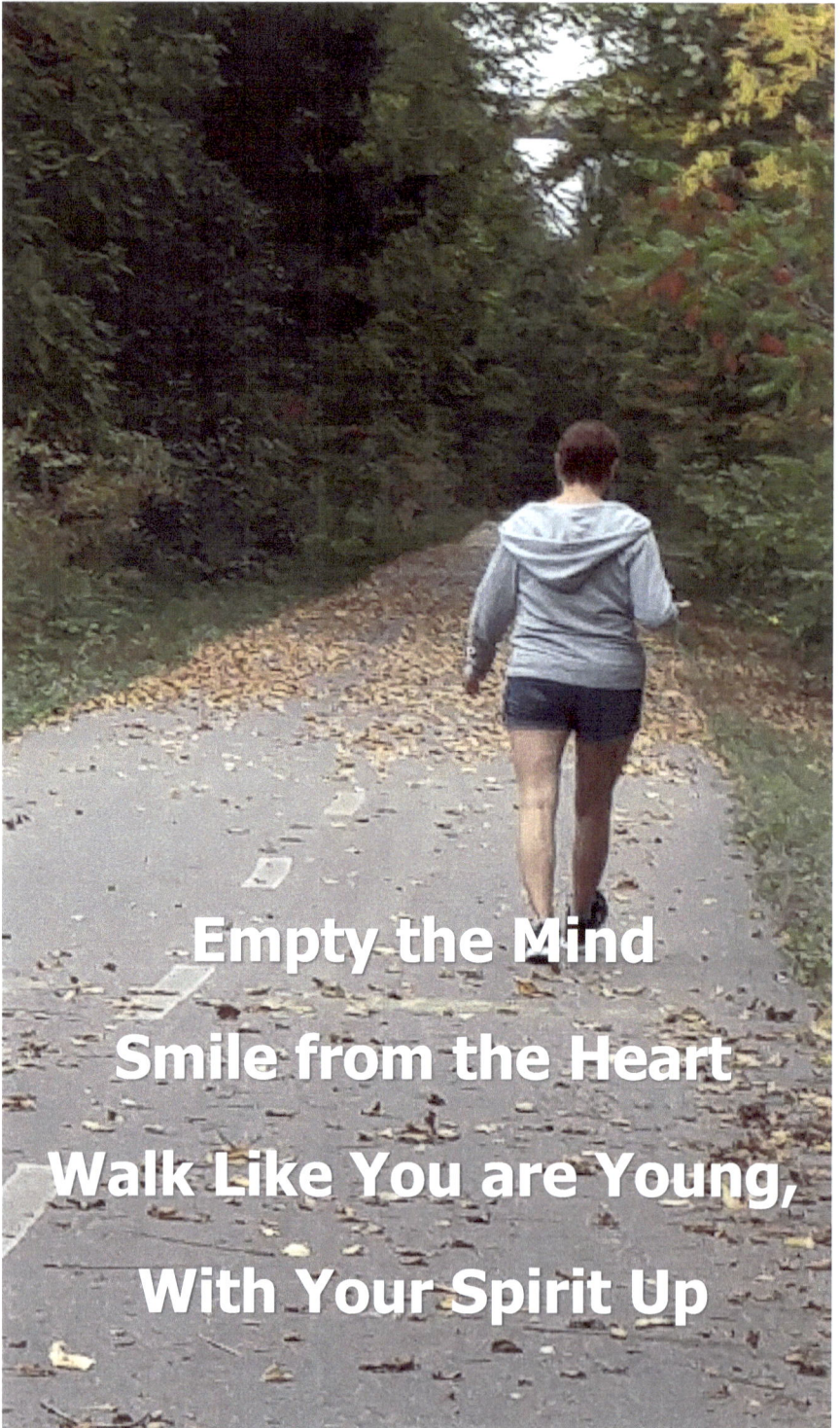

Empty the Mind

Smile from the Heart

Walk Like You are Young,

With Your Spirit Up

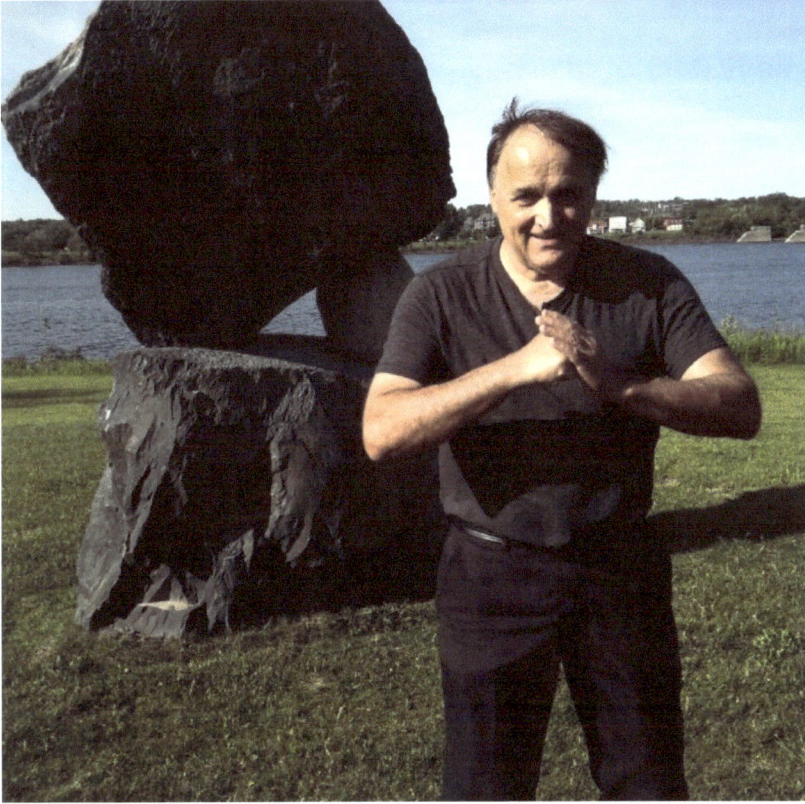

Authors' Note

The core information in this book has been gathered from training I received over the last 22 years from my two Qi Gong teachers as well as from my training in Massage Therapy, Healing Touch, and Acupuncture.

I am not a Medical Doctor. The exercises and information found in this book are not intended to replace personalized medical care or treatment. If you have any doubt about your ability to practice Qi Gong or to do Qi Healing, please consult with your physician.

Benefits from practicing Qi Gong vary from person to person. For the best results, cultivate a positive spirit, and follow a healthy diet and lifestyle. Persons suffering from mental illness or epilepsy should refrain from practice Qi Gong.

References

A Brief History of Qi - Zhang Yu Huan & Ken Rose - Paradigm Publications, 2001

A Manual of Acupuncture - Peter Deadman & Mazin Al-Khafaji - Journal of Chinese Medicine Publications, 2007

Anatomy of the Spirit - Caroline Myss, Three Rivers Press, New York, 1996

Acupressure's Potent Points - Michael Reed Gach – Bantam Books, 1990

Chinese Medical Qi Gong Therapy - Dr. Jerry Alan Johnson - International Institute of Qi Gong, 2000

Chinese Medical Qigong Therapy - Grand Master Tzu Kuo Shih, OMD, L.Ac., and Melanie Shih, OMD, L.Ac. - Second Military Medical University Press, 2010

Chinese Medical Qi Gong - Tianjun Liu, O.M.D. & Kevin Chen, Ph.D. - Singing Dragon 2010

Chinese Martial Arts - The Teachings of Grandmaster Cai Song Fang by Jan Diepersloot. 1995

Chi Kung: Way of Power by Master Lam Kam Chuen. Human Kinetics 2003

Dream Healer - Adam, Penguin Canada, 2003

Foundations of Chinese Medicine - Giovanni Maciocia, Elsevier, 2005

Healing Touch, A Guidebook for Practitioners - Dorothea Hover-Kramer, Delmar Tomson Learning, 2002

Ki in Daily Life by Koichi Tohei. Seiwa Printing 1978

Life More Abundant - Xiaoguang Jin and Joseph Marcello - Buy Books on the Web.Com, 1999

Living Pain Free with Acupressure - Dr. Devi S. Nambudripad, 1997

Qi Gong Empowerment: A Guide to Medical, Taoist, Buddhist & Wushu Energy Cultivation by Master Shou-Yu Liang & Wen-Ching Wu. Way of the Dragon Publishing, USA 1997

Qi Gong Therapy by Tzu Kuo Shih, Station Hill, 1994

The Chinese Art of Healing with Energy - Qi Gong Therapy - Dr. Tsu Kuo Shih, Station Hill Press, 1994

The Art of Peace - Moreihei Ueshiba, Shambhala, 1992

The Qi Gong Workbook for Anxiety by Master Kam Chuen Lam, New Harbinger Publications Inc,2014

The Essence of Shaolin White Crane - Martial Power & Qi Gong by Dr. Jwing-Ming Yang. YMAA Publications 1996

The Mysterious Power of Ki - The Force Within by Kouzo Kaku, Global Books Limited 2000

The Swimming Dragon by Tzu Kuo Shih, Station Hill Press, 1989

T'ai Chi Ch'uan for Health & Self-Defense by Master T.T. Liang, Redwing Book Company, Boston, 1974

Wudang Qigong - Yuzeng Liu - International Wudang Internal Martial Arts Research Association, 1999

Warriors of Stillness: Meditative Traditions in the Chinese Martial Arts - The Teachings of Grandmaster Cai Song Fang by Jan Diepersloot. 1995